Easy Mediterranean Soups & Salads

50 Unmissable Soup & Salad Recipes for Your Mediterranean Meals

Carmen Berlanti

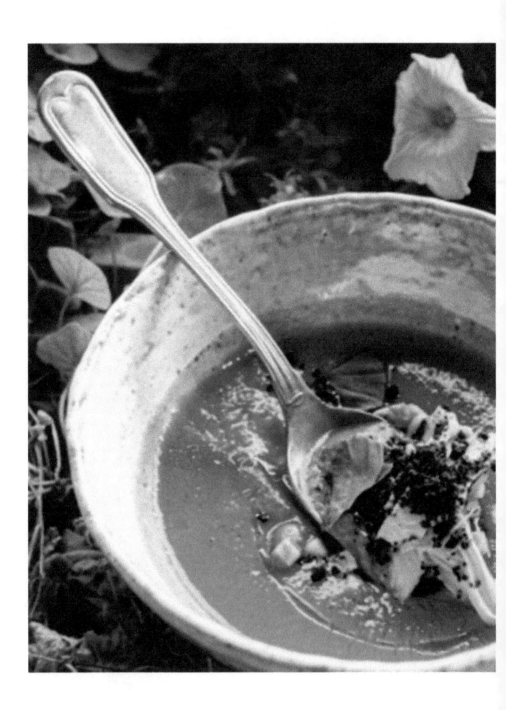

Table of Contents

PORK AND GREENS SALAD 6

MEDITERRANEAN DUCK BREAST SALAD 8

MEDITERRANEAN CHICKEN BITES 11

MEDITERRANEAN CHICKEN AND TOMATO DISH 13

CREAMY CHICKEN SALAD 15

CHICKEN AND CABBAGE MIX 17

CHICKEN AND QUINOA SALAD 19

SIMPLE PORK STIR FRY 21

BEEF TARTAR 24

MELON SALAD 26

ORANGE CELERY SALAD 28

ROASTED BROCCOLI SALAD 30

TOMATO SALAD 33

FETA BEET SALAD 35

CAULIFLOWER & TOMATO SALAD 36

TAHINI SPINACH 38

PILAF WITH CREAM CHEESE 40

EASY SPAGHETTI SQUASH 42

PISTACHIO ARUGULA SALAD 44

PENNE WITH TAHINI SAUCE 46

ROASTED VEGGIES 48

ZUCCHINI PASTA 50

ASPARAGUS PASTA 52

FETA & SPINACH PITA BAKE 54

CHEESY CAPRESE SALAD SKEWERS 56

ANDALUSIAN GAZPACHO 58

TABBOULEH SALAD 61

FATTOUSH 63

ALMOST NIÇOISE SALAD... 66

MEDITERRANEAN POTATO SALAD 68

PANZANELLA SALAD.. 70

LENTIL AND FETA SALAD.. 73

GREEK SALAD... 75

SHEPHERD'S SALAD 78

SPANISH GREEN BEANS 80

RUSTIC CAULIFLOWER AND CARROT HASH 82

ROASTED CAULIFLOWER AND TOMATOES 84

SAUTÉED GARLIC SPINACH 86

GARLICKY SAUTÉED ZUCCHINI WITH MINT 89

STEWED OKRA... 91

FAVA AND GARBANZO BEAN FŪL 93

CONFETTI COUSCOUS 95

LEMON ORZO WITH FRESH HERBS... 97

ORZO-VEGGIE PILAF.. 99

BULGUR AND GARBANZO PILAF 101

SPANISH RICE.. 103

GARBANZO AND PITA NO-BAKE CASSEROLE 105

QUICK SHRIMP FETTUCCINE 107

WHITE PIZZA WITH PROSCIUTTO AND ARUGULA 110

Pork and Greens Salad

Difficulty Level: 2/5

Preparation time: 10 minutes

Cooking time: 15 minutes

Servings: 4

Ingredients:

1 pound pork chops, boneless and cut into strips

8 ounces white mushrooms, sliced

½ cup Italian dressing

6 cups mixed salad greens

6 ounces jarred artichoke hearts, drained

Salt and black pepper to the taste

½ cup basil, chopped

1 tablespoon olive oil

Directions:

Heat a pan with the oil over medium-high heat, add the pork and brown for 5 minutes.

Add the mushrooms, stir and sauté for 5 minutes more.

Add the dressing, artichokes, salad greens, salt, pepper and the basil, cook for 4-5 minutes, divide everything into bowls and serve.

Nutrition:

Calories: 235

Fat: 6g

Fiber: 4g

Carbohydrates: 14g

Protein: 11g

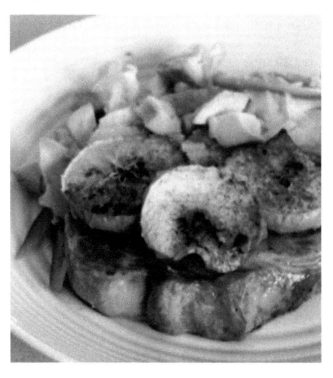

Mediterranean Duck Breast Salad

Difficulty Level: 2/5

Preparation time: 10 minutes

Cooking time: **20 minutes**

Servings: 4

Ingredients:

3 tablespoons white wine vinegar

2 tablespoons sugar

2 oranges, peeled and cut into segments

1 teaspoon orange zest, grated

1 tablespoons lemon juice

1 teaspoon lemon zest, grated

3 tablespoons shallot, minced

tablespoons canola oil

Salt and black pepper to taste

2 duck breasts, boneless but skin on, cut into 4 pieces

1 head of frisée, torn

2 small lettuce heads washed, torn into small pieces

2 tablespoons chives, chopped

Directions:

Heat a small saucepan over medium high heat, add vinegar and sugar, stir and boil for 5 minutes and take off heat.

Add orange zest, lemon zest and lemon juice, stir and leave aside for a few minutes. Add shallot, salt and pepper to taste and the oil, whisk well and leave aside for now.

Pat dry duck pieces, score skin, trim and season with salt and pepper. Heat a pan over medium high heat for 1 minute, arrange duck breast pieces skin side down, brown for 8 minutes, reduce heat to medium and cook for 4 more minutes.

Flip pieces, cook for 3 minutes, transfer to a cutting board and cover them with foil. Put frisée and lettuce in a bowl, stir and divide between plates.

Slice duck, arrange on top, add orange segments, sprinkle chives and drizzle the vinaigrette.

Nutrition:

Calories: 320

Fat: 4g

Fiber: 4g

Carbohydrates: 6g

Protein: 14g

Mediterranean Chicken Bites

Difficulty Level: 2/5

Preparation time: 10 minutes

Cooking time: **10 minutes**

Servings: 4

Ingredients:

20 ounces canned pineapple slices

A drizzle of olive oil

3 cups chicken thighs, boneless, skinless and cut into medium pieces

A tablespoon of smoked paprika

Directions:

Heat a pan over medium high heat, add pineapple slices, cook them for a few minutes on each side, transfer to a cutting board, cool them down and cut into medium cubes.

Heat another pan with a drizzle of oil over medium high heat, rub chicken pieces with paprika, add them to the pan and cook for 5 minutes on each side.

Arrange chicken cubes on a platter, add a pineapple piece on top of each and stick a toothpick in each, and serve.

Nutrition:

Calories: 120

Fat: 3g

Fiber: 1g

Carbohydrates: 5g

Protein: 2g

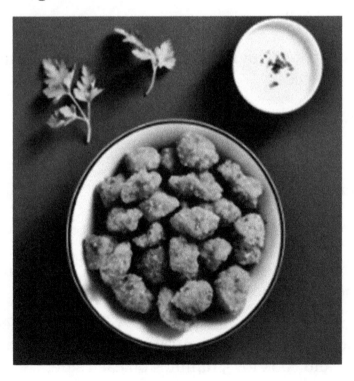

Mediterranean Chicken And Tomato Dish

Difficulty Level: 2/5

Preparation time: **10 minutes**

Cooking time: **20 minutes**

Servings: 4

Ingredients:

Chicken thighs

A tablespoon of olive oil

1 Tablespoon thyme, chopped

Garlic cloves, minced

1 Teaspoon red pepper flakes, crushed

½ cup heavy cream

¾ cup chicken stock

½ cup sun dried tomatoes in olive oil, drained and chopped

Salt and black pepper to taste

¼ cup parmesan cheese, grated

Basil leaves, chopped for serving

Directions:

Heat a pan with the oil over medium high heat, add chicken, salt and pepper to taste, cook for 3 minutes on each side, transfer to a plate and leave aside for now.

Return pan to heat, add thyme, garlic and pepper flakes, stir and cook for 1 minute.

Add stock, tomatoes, salt and pepper, heavy cream and parmesan, stir and bring to a simmer.

Add chicken pieces, stir, place in the oven at 350 degrees F and bake for 15 minutes.

Take pan out of the oven, leave chicken aside for 2-3 minutes, divide between plates and serve with basil sprinkled on top.

Nutrition:

Calories: 212

Fat: 4g

Fiber: 3g

Carbohydrates: 3g

Protein: 3g

Creamy Chicken Salad

Difficulty Level: 1/5

Preparation time: 10 minutes

Servings: 6

Ingredients:

20 ounces chicken meat, already cooked and chopped

½ cup pecans, chopped

1 cup green grapes, seedless and cut in halves

½ cup celery, chopped

2 ounces canned mandarin oranges, drained

For the creamy cucumber salad dressing:

1 cup Greek yogurt cucumber, chopped garlic clove, chopped

Salt and white pepper to taste

1 teaspoon lemon juice

Directions:

In a bowl, mix cucumber with salt, pepper to taste, lemon juice, garlic and yogurt and stir very well.

In a salad bowl, mix chicken meat with grapes, pecans, oranges and celery.

Add cucumber salad dressing, toss to coat and keep in the fridge until you serve it.

Nutrition:

Calories: 200

Fat: 3g

Fiber: 1g

Carbohydrates: 2g

Protein: 8g

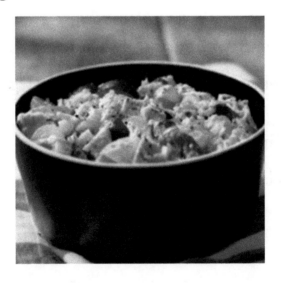

Chicken and Cabbage Mix

Difficulty Level: 2/5

Preparation time: 10 minutes

Cooking time: **6 minutes**

Servings: 4

Ingredients:

3 medium chicken breasts, skinless, boneless and cut into thin strips

4 ounces green cabbage, shredded

5 tablespoon extra virgin olive oil

Salt and black pepper to taste

2 tablespoons sherry vinegar tablespoon chives, chopped

¼ cup feta cheese, crumbled

¼ cup barbeque sauce

Bacon slices, cooked and crumbled

Directions:

In a bowl, mix 4 tablespoon oil with vinegar, salt and pepper to taste and stir well.

Add the shredded cabbage, toss to coat and leave aside for now.

Season chicken with salt and pepper, heat a pan with remaining oil over medium high heat, add chicken, cook for 6 minutes, take off heat, transfer to a bowl and mix well with barbeque sauce.

Arrange salad on serving plates, add chicken strips, sprinkle cheese, chives and crumbled bacon and serve right away.

Nutrition:

Calories: 200

Fat: 15g

Fiber: 3g

Carbohydrates: 10g

Protein: 33g

Chicken and Quinoa Salad

Difficulty Level: 2/5

Preparation time: 10 minutes

Cooking time: **20 minutes**

Servings: 2

Ingredients:

2 tablespoons olive oil

2 ounces quinoa

2 ounces cherry tomatoes, cut in quarters

3 ounces sweet corn

A handful coriander, chopped

Lime juice from 1 lime

Lime zest from 1 lime, grated

Salt and black pepper to taste

2 spring onions, chopped

Small red chilli pepper, chopped

Avocado, pitted, peeled and chopped

2 ounces chicken meat, roasted, skinless, boneless and chopped

Directions:

Put some water in a pan, bring to a boil over medium high heat, add quinoa, stir and cook for 12 minutes.

Meanwhile, put corn in a pan, heat over medium high heat, cook for 5 minutes and leave aside for now.

Drain quinoa, transfer to a bowl, add tomatoes, corn, coriander, onions, chilli, lime zest, olive oil, salt and black pepper to taste and toss.

In another bowl, mix avocado with lime juice and stir well.

Add this to quinoa salad, and chicken, toss to coat and serve.

Nutrition:

Calories: 320

Fat: 4g

Fiber: 4g

Carbohydrates: 5g

Protein: 7g

Simple Pork Stir Fry

Difficulty Level: 2/5

Preparation time: 10 minutes

Cooking time: **15 minutes**

Servings: 4

Ingredients:

4 ounces bacon, chopped

4 ounces snow peas

2 tablespoons butter

1 pound pork loin, cut into thin strips

2 cups mushrooms, sliced

¾ cup white wine

½ cup yellow onion, chopped

3 tablespoons sour cream

Salt and white pepper to taste

Directions:

Put snow peas in a saucepan, add water to cover, add a pinch of salt, bring to a boil over medium heat, cook until they are soft, drain and leave aside.

Heat a pan over medium high heat, add bacon, cook for a few minutes, drain grease, transfer to a bowl and also leave aside.

Heat a pan with 1 tablespoon butter over medium heat, add pork strips, salt and pepper to taste, brown for a few minutes and transfer to a plate as well.

Return pan to medium heat, add remaining butter and melt it. Add onions and mushrooms, stir and cook for 4 minutes.

Add wine, and simmer until it's reduced. Add cream, peas, pork, salt and pepper to taste, stir, heat up, divide between plates, top with bacon and serve.

Nutrition:

Calories: 310

Fat: 4g

Fiber: 6g

Carbohydrates: 9g

Protein: 10g

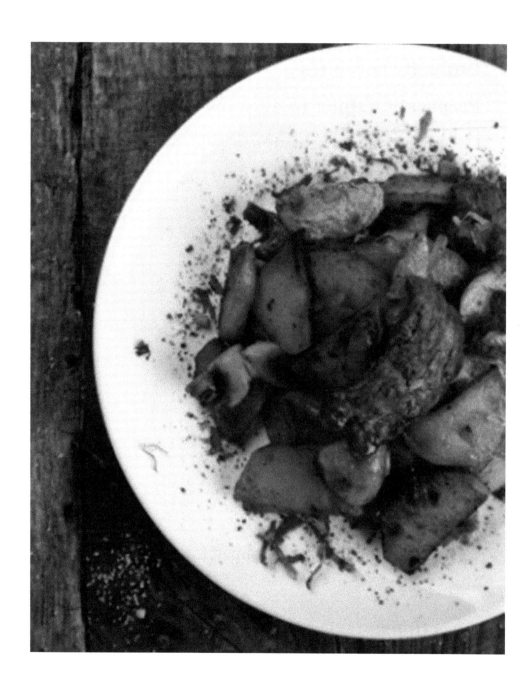

Beef Tartar

Difficulty Level: 1/5

Preparation time: 10 minutes

Cooking time: 0 minutes

Servings: 1

Ingredients:

1 shallot, chopped

4 ounces beef fillet, minced

5 small cucumbers, chopped

1 egg yolk

A pinch of salt and black pepper

2 teaspoons mustard

1 tablespoon parsley, chopped

1 parsley spring, roughly chopped for serving

Directions:

In a bowl, mix meat with shallot, egg yolk, salt, pepper, mustard, cucumbers and parsley.

Stir well and arrange on a platter.

Garnish with the chopped parsley spring and serve.

Nutrition:

Calories: 210

Fat: 3g

Fiber: 1g

Carbohydrates: 5g

Protein: 8g

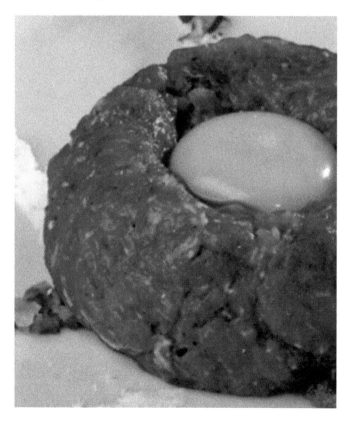

Melon Salad

Difficulty Level: 1/5

Preparation time: 20 Minutes

Cooking time: 0 minutes

Servings: 6

Ingredients:

¼ teaspoon sea salt

¼ teaspoon black pepper

1 tablespoon balsamic vinegar

1 cantaloupe, quartered & seeded

12 watermelons, small & seedless

2 cups mozzarella balls, fresh

1/3 cup basil, fresh & torn

2 tablespoons olive oil

Directions:

Get out a melon baller and scoop out balls of cantaloupe, and the put them in a colander over a serving bowl.

Use your melon baller to cut the watermelon as well, and then put them in with your cantaloupe.

Allow your fruit to drain for ten minutes, and then refrigerate the juice for another recipe. It can even be added to smoothies.

Wipe the bowl dry, and then place your fruit in it.

Add in your basil, oil, vinegar, mozzarella and tomatoes before seasoning with salt and pepper.

Gently mix and serve immediately or chilled.

Nutrition:

Calories: 218

Protein: 10g

Fat: 13g

Carbohydrates: 17g

Orange Celery Salad

Difficulty Level: 1/5
Preparation time: 15 Minutes
Cooking time: 0 minutes
Servings: 6

Ingredients:

1 tablespoon lemon juice, fresh

¼ teaspoon sea salt, fine

¼ teaspoon black pepper

1 tablespoon olive brine

1 tablespoon olive oil

¼ cup red onion, sliced

½ cup green olives

2 oranges, peeled & sliced

3 celery stalks, sliced diagonally in ½ inch slices

Directions:

Put your oranges, olives, onion and celery in a shallow bowl.

In a different bowl whisk your oil, olive brine and lemon juice, pour this over your salad.

Season with salt and pepper before serving.

Nutrition:

Calories: 65

Protein: 2g

Fat: 0g

Carbohydrates: 9g

Roasted Broccoli Salad

Difficulty Level: 2/5

Preparation time: 10 Minutes

Cooking time: 20 minutes

Servings: 4

Ingredients:

1 lb. Broccoli, cut into florets & stem sliced

3 tablespoons olive oil, divided

1 pint cherry tomatoes

1 1/2 teaspoons honey, raw & divided

3 cups cubed bread, whole grain

1 tablespoon balsamic vinegar

1/2 teaspoon black pepper

1/4 teaspoon sea salt, fine

Grated parmesan for serving

Directions:

Start by heating your oven to 450, and then get out a rimmed baking sheet. Place it in the oven to heat up.

Drizzle your broccoli with a tablespoon of oil, and toss to coat.

Remove the baking sheet form the oven, and spoon the broccoli on it. Leave oil it eh bottom of the bowl and add in your tomatoes, toss to coat, and then toss your tomatoes with a tablespoon of honey. Pour them on the same baking sheet as your broccoli.

Roast for fifteen minutes, and stir halfway through your cooking time.

Add in your bread, and then roast for three more minutes.

Whisk two tablespoons of oil, vinegar, and remaining honey. Season with salt and pepper. Pour this over your broccoli mix to serve.

Nutrition:

Calories: 226

Protein: 7g

Fat: 12g

Carbohydrates: 26g

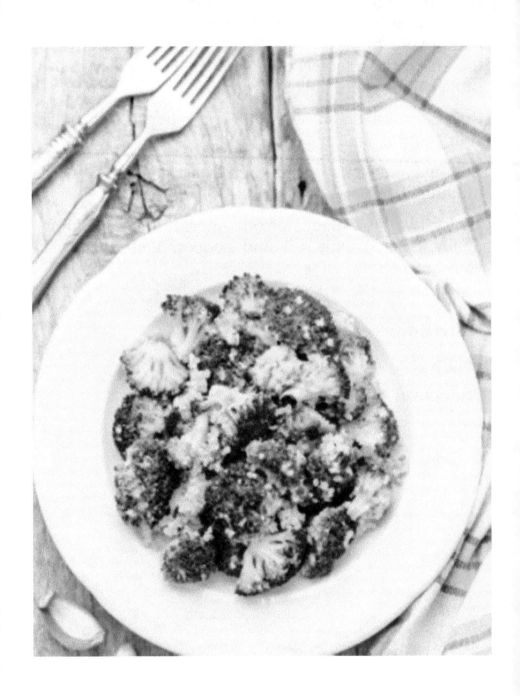

Tomato Salad

Difficulty Level: 1/5

Preparation time: 20 Minutes

Cooking time: 0 minutes

Servings: *4*

Ingredients:

1 cucumber, sliced

¼ cup sun dried tomatoes, chopped

1 lb. Tomatoes, cubed

½ cup black olives

1 red onion, sliced

1 tablespoon balsamic vinegar

¼ cup parsley, fresh & chopped

2 tablespoons olive oil

Sea salt & black pepper to taste

Directions:

Get out a bowl and combine all of your vegetables together. To make your dressing mix all your seasoning, olive oil and vinegar.

Toss with your salad and serve fresh.

Nutrition:

Calories: 126

Protein: 2.1g

Fat: 9.2g

Carbohydrates: 11.5g

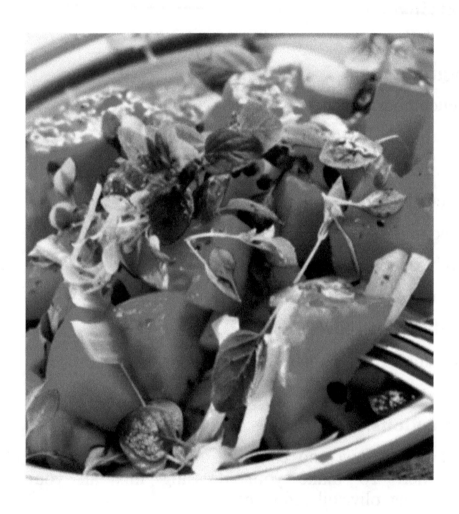

Feta Beet Salad

Difficulty Level: 1/5

Preparation time: 15 Minutes

Cooking time: 0 minutes

Servings: *4*

Ingredients:

6 red beets, cooked & peeled

3 ounces feta cheese, cubed

2 tablespoons olive oil

2 tablespoons balsamic vinegar

Directions:

Combine everything together, and then serve.

Nutrition:

Calories: 230

Protein: 7.3g

Fat: 12g

Carbohydrates: 26.3g

Cauliflower & Tomato Salad

Difficulty Level: 1/5

Preparation time: 15 Minutes

Cooking time: 0 minutes

Servings: 4

Ingredients:

1 head cauliflower, chopped

2 tablespoons parsley, fresh & chopped

2 cups cherry tomatoes, halved

2 tablespoons lemon juice, fresh

2 tablespoons pine nuts

Sea salt & black pepper to taste

Directions:

Mix your lemon juice, cherry tomatoes, cauliflower and parsley together, and then season. Top with pine nuts, and mix well before serving.

Nutrition:

Calories: 64

Protein: 2.8g

Fat: 3.3g

Carbohydrates: 7.9g

Tahini Spinach

Difficulty Level: 2/5

Preparation time: 15 Minutes

Cooking time: 5 Minutes

Servings: *3*

Ingredients:

10 spinach, chopped

½ cup water

1 tablespoon tahini

2 cloves garlic, minced

¼ teaspoon cumin

¼ teaspoon paprika

¼ teaspoon cayenne pepper

1/3 cup red wine vinegar

Sea salt & black pepper to taste

Directions:

Add your spinach and water to the saucepan, and then boil it on high heat. Once boiling reduce to low, and cover. Allow it to cook on simmer for five minutes.

Add in your garlic, cumin, cayenne, red wine vinegar, paprika and tahini. Whisk well, and season with salt and pepper.

Drain your spinach and top with tahini sauce to serve.

Nutrition:

Calories: 69

Protein: 5g

Fat: 3g

Carbohydrates: 8g

Pilaf with Cream Cheese

Difficulty Level: 2/5

Preparation time: 0 Minutes

Cooking time: 25 minutes

Servings: 6

Ingredients:

2 cups yellow long grain rice, parboiled

1 cup onion

4 green onions

3 tablespoons butter

3 tablespoons vegetable broth

2 teaspoons cayenne pepper

1 teaspoons paprika

½ teaspoon cloves, minced

2 tablespoons mint leaves, fresh & chopped

1 bunch fresh mint leaves to garnish

1 tablespoons olive oil

Sea salt & black pepper to taste

Cheese cream:

3 tablespoons olive oil

Sea salt & black pepper to taste

9 ounces cream cheese

Directions:

Start by heating your oven to 360, and then get out a pan. Heat your butter and olive oil together, and cook your onions and spring onions for two minutes.

Add in your salt, pepper, paprika, cloves, vegetable broth, rice and remaining seasoning. S

Sauté for three minutes.

Cover with foil, and bake for another half hour. Allow it to cool.

Mix in the cream cheese, cheese, olive oil, salt and pepper. Serve your pilaf garnished with fresh mint leaves.

Nutrition:

Calories: 364

Protein: 5g

Fat: 30g

Carbohydrates: 20g

Easy Spaghetti Squash

Difficulty Level: 3/5

Preparation time: 5 Minutes

Cooking time: 25 minutes

Servings: 6

Ingredients:

2 spring onions, chopped fine

3 cloves garlic, minced

1 zucchini, diced

1 red bell pepper, diced

1 tablespoon Italian seasoning

1 tomato, small & chopped fine

1 tablespoons parsley, fresh & chopped

Pinch lemon pepper

Dash sea salt, fine

4 ounces feta cheese, crumbled

3 Italian sausage links, casing removed

2 tablespoons olive oil

1 spaghetti sauce, halved lengthwise

Directions:

Start by heating your oven to 350, and get out a large baking sheet. Coat it with cooking spray, and then put your squash on it with the cut side down.

Bake at 350 for forty-five minutes. It should be tender.

Turn the squash over, and bake for five more minutes. Scrape the strands into a larger bowl.

Heat up a tablespoon of olive oil in a skillet, and then add in your Italian sausage. Cook at eight minutes before removing it and placing it in a bowl.

Add another tablespoon of olive oil to the skillet and cook your garlic and onions until softened. This will take five minutes. Throw in your Italian seasoning, red peppers and zucchini. Cook for another five minutes. Your vegetables should be softened.

Mix in your feta cheese and squash, cooking until the cheese has melted.

Stir in your sausage, and then season with lemon pepper and salt. Serve with parsley and tomato.

Nutrition:

Calories: 423

Protein: 18g

Fat: 30g

Carbohydrates: 22g

Pistachio Arugula Salad

Difficulty Level: 1/5

Preparation time: 20 Minutes

Cooking time: 0 minutes

Serves: 6

Ingredients:

6 cups kale, chopped

¼ cup olive oil

2 tablespoons lemon juice, fresh

½ teaspoon smoked paprika

2 cups arugula

1/3 cup pistachios, unsalted & shelled

6 tablespoons parmesan cheese, grated

Directions:

Get a salad bowl and combine your oil, lemon, smoked paprika and kale. Gently massage the leaves for half a minute. Your kale should be coated well.

Gently mix your arugula and pistachios when ready to serve.

Nutrition:

Calories: 150

Protein: 5g

Fat: 12g

Carbohydrates: 8g

Penne with Tahini Sauce

Difficulty Level: 2/5

Preparation time: 5 Minutes

Cooking time: 15 minutes

Serves: 8

Ingredients:

1/3 cup water

1 cup yogurt, plain

1/8 cup lemon juice

3 tablespoons tahini

3 cloves garlic

1 onion, chopped

¼ cup olive oil

2 Portobello mushrooms, large & sliced

½ red bell pepper, diced

16 ounces penne pasta

½ cup parsley, fresh & chopped

Black pepper to taste

Directions:

Start by getting out a pot and bring a pot of salted water to a boil. Cook your pasta al dente per package instructions.

Mix your lemon juice and tahini together, and then place it tin a food processor. Process with garlic, water and yogurt. It should be smooth.

Get out a saucepan, and place it over medium heat. Heat up your oil, and cook your onions until soft.

Add in your mushroom and continue to cook until softened.

Add in your bell pepper, and cook until crispy.

Drain your pasta, and then toss with your tahini sauce, top with parsley and pepper and serve with vegetables.

Nutrition:

Calories: 332

Proteins: 11g

Fat: 12g

Carbohydrates: 48g

Roasted Veggies

Difficulty Level: 2/5

Preparation time: 5 Minutes

Cooking time: 25 minutes

Serves: *12*

Ingredients:

6 cloves garlic

6 tablespoons olive oil

1 fennel bulb, diced

1 zucchini, diced

2 red bell peppers, diced

6 potatoes, large & diced

2 teaspoons sea salt

½ cup balsamic vinegar

¼ cup rosemary, chopped & fresh

2 teaspoons vegetable bouillon powder

Directions:

Start by heating your oven to 400.

Get out a baking dish and place your potatoes, fennel, zucchini, garlic and fennel on a baking dish, drizzling with olive oil. Sprinkle with salt, bouillon powder, and rosemary. Mix well, and then bake at 450 for thirty to forty minutes. Mix your vinegar into the vegetables before serving.

Nutrition:

Calories: 675

Protein: 13g

Fat: 21g

Carbohydrates: 112g

Zucchini Pasta

Difficulty Level: 2/5

Preparation time: 10 Minutes

Cooking time: 20 minutes

Servings: 4

Ingredients:

3 tablespoons olive oil

2 cloves garlic, minced

3 zucchini, large & diced

Sea salt & black pepper to taste

½ cup milk, 2%

¼ teaspoon nutmeg

1 tablespoon lemon juice, fresh

½ cup parmesan, grated

8 ounces uncooked farfalle pasta

Directions:

Get out a skillet and place it over medium heat, and then heat up the oil. Add in your garlic and cook for a minute. Stir often so that it doesn't burn. Add in your salt, pepper and zucchini. Stir well, and cook covered for fifteen minutes. During this time, you'll want to stir the mixture twice.

Get out a microwave safe bowl, and heat the milk for thirty seconds. Stir in your nutmeg, and then pour it into the skillet. Cook uncovered for five minutes. Stir occasionally to keep from burning.

Get out a stockpot and cook your pasta per package instructions. Drain the pasta, and then save two tablespoons of pasta water.

Stir everything together, and add in the cheese and lemon juice and pasta water.

Nutrition:

Calories: 410

Protein: 15g

Fat: 17g

Carbohydrates: 45g

Asparagus Pasta

Difficulty Level: 2/5

Preparation time: 10 Minutes

Cooking time: 15 minutes

Serves: 6

Ingredients:

8 ounces farfalle pasta, uncooked

1 ½ cups asparagus, fresh, trimmed & chopped into 1 inch pieces

1 pint grape tomatoes, halved

2 tablespoons olive oil

Sea salt & black pepper to taste

2 cups mozzarella, fresh & drained

1/3 cup basil leaves, fresh & torn

2 tablespoons balsamic vinegar

Directions:

Start by heating the oven to 400, and then get out a stockpot. Cook your pasta per package instructions, and reserve ¼ cup of pasta water.

Get out a bowl and toss the tomatoes, oil, asparagus, and season with salt and pepper. Spread this mixture on a baking sheet, and bake for fifteen minutes. Stir twice in this time.

Remove your vegetables from the oven, and then add the cooked pasta to your baking sheet. Mix with a few tablespoons of pasta water so that your sauce becomes smoother.

Mix in your basil and mozzarella, drizzling with balsamic vinegar. Serve warm.

Nutrition:

Calories: 307

Protein: 18g

Fat: 14g

Carbohydrates: 33g

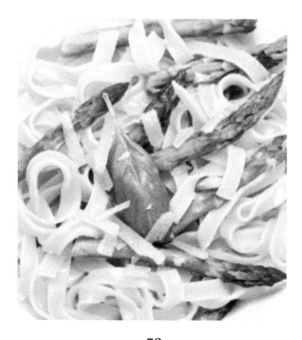

Feta & Spinach Pita Bake

Difficulty Level: 2/5

Preparation time: 10 Minutes

Cooking time: 15 minutes

Serves: 6

Ingredients:

2 Roma tomatoes, chopped

6 whole wheat pita bread

1 jar sun dried tomato pesto

4 mushrooms, fresh & sliced

1 bunch spinach, rinsed & chopped

2 tablespoons parmesan cheese, grated

3 tablespoons olive oil

½ cup feta cheese, crumbled

Dash black pepper

Directions:

Start by heating the oven to 350, and get to your pita bread. Spread the tomato pesto on the side of each one. Put them in a baking pan with the tomato side up.

Top with tomatoes, spinach, mushrooms, parmesan and feta. Drizzle with olive oil and season with pepper.

Bake for twelve minutes, and then serve cut into quarters.

Nutrition:

Calories: 350

Protein: 12g

Fat: 17g

Carbohydrates: 42g

Cheesy Caprese Salad Skewers

Difficulty Level: 1/5

Preparation time: 15 minutes

Cooking time: 0 minutes

Servings: 10

Ingredients:

8-oz cherry tomatoes, sliced in half

A handful of fresh basil leaves, rinsed and drained

1-lb fresh mozzarella, cut into bite-sized slices

Balsamic vinegar

Extra virgin olive oil

Freshly ground black pepper

Toothpicks

Directions:

Sandwich a folded basil leaf and mozzarella cheese between the halves of tomato onto a toothpick.

Drizzle with olive oil and balsamic vinegar each skewer. To serve, sprinkle with freshly ground black pepper.

Nutrition:

Calories: 94

Total Fats: 3.7g

Fiber: 2g

Carbohydrates: 15.4g

Protein: 2.1g

Andalusian Gazpacho

Difficulty Level: 1/5

Preparation time: 20 minutes

Cooking time: 0 minutes

Servings: 10

Ingredients:

2 slices slightly stale bread, crusts removed

2 small cucumbers, peeled and finely chopped, divided

1 small sweet onion, finely chopped

1 garlic clove, mashed

3 pounds ripe tomatoes, peeled, seeded, and diced, plus 1 tomato, finely diced

1 green bell pepper, seeded and diced

3 tablespoons red wine vinegar

6 tablespoons olive oil

1 teaspoon chopped fresh oregano

⅛ teaspoon salt

⅛ teaspoon freshly ground black pepper

4 scallions, white and green parts, chopped

Directions:

In a shallow bowl, combine the bread with enough water to cover. Soak the bread for about 2 minutes until just softened. Squeeze out the excess water and place the bread in a food processor.

Add half the cucumbers, the onion, garlic, and diced tomatoes to the food processor. Purée until smooth and transfer to a large bowl.

Stir in the remaining cucumbers, green bell pepper, and vinegar.

In a small bowl, stir together the olive oil, finely diced tomato, oregano, salt, and pepper.

Divide the soup evenly among bowls and sprinkle with the tomato-pepper mixture and scallions.

Nutrition:

Calories: 215

Total Fats: 15g

Fiber: 2g

Carbohydrates: 20g

Protein: 4g

Sodium: 111mg

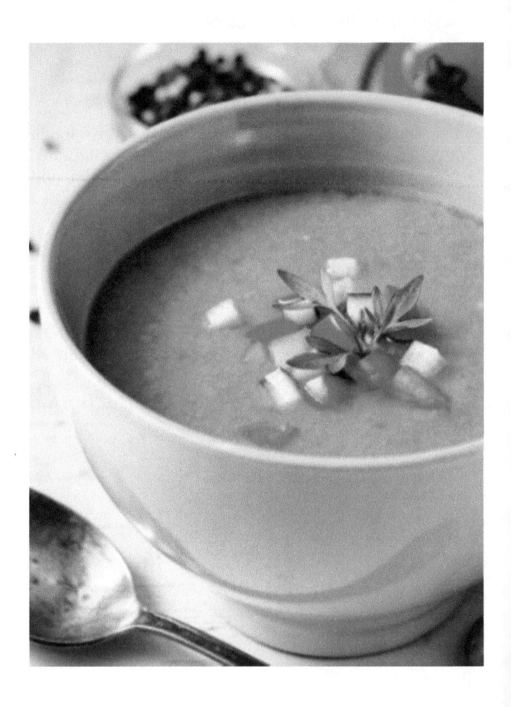

Tabbouleh Salad

Difficulty Level: 1/5

Preparation time: 20 minutes

Cooking time: 0 minutes

Servings: 6

Ingredients:

1 cup fine bulgur wheat

1 cup hot water

4 cups finely chopped fresh parsley

2 tomatoes, diced

1 sweet onion, chopped

½ cup olive oil

½ cup freshly squeezed lemon juice, plus more as needed

⅛ teaspoon salt, plus more as needed

Directions:

In a medium bowl, combine the bulgur and hot water. Let sit for about 5 minutes until soft.

In another medium bowl, stir together the parsley, tomatoes, and onion.

Drain the excess water from the bulgur and add it to the tomato mixture.

Drizzle with the olive oil and lemon juice. Stir to combine. Sprinkle with the salt, taste, and add more salt or lemon juice, as needed.

Refrigerate leftovers in an airtight container for up to 1 week.

SUBSTITUTION TIP: For people allergic to gluten, replace the bulgur with cooked quinoa.

Nutrition:

Calories: 260

Total Fats: 18g

Saturated Fat: 3g

Fiber: 5g

Carbohydrates: 23g

Protein: 5g

Sodium: 82mg

Fattoush

Difficulty Level: 2/5

Preparation time: 20 minutes

Cooking time: 5 minutes

Servings: 6

Ingredients:

2 loaves slightly stale pita bread, cut into 2-inch squares

½ cup olive oil

¼ cup freshly squeezed lemon juice

2 tablespoons pomegranate molasses, or cranberry juice

1 tablespoon Sanaa's Za'atar, or store-bought

6 romaine lettuce leaves, chopped

2 tomatoes, diced

2 Persian cucumbers, diced

1 red bell pepper, seeded and diced

4 scallions, white and green parts, chopped

2 radishes, thinly sliced

1 cup chopped fresh parsley

½ cup chopped fresh mint

Salt

Freshly ground black pepper

Directions:

Preheat the oven to 350°F.

Place the pita squares in a single layer on a baking sheet and toast in the oven for about 5 minutes until golden. Remove and set aside.

In a medium bowl, whisk the olive oil, lemon juice, molasses, and za'atar until blended. Set aside.

In a large bowl, combine the lettuce, tomatoes, cucumbers, red bell pepper, scallions, radishes, parsley, and mint. Drizzle with the dressing and toss well to coat. Taste and season with salt and pepper, as needed. Top with the pita chips to serve.

Nutrition:

Calories: 253

Total Fats: 18g

Saturated Fat: 3g

Fiber: 5g

Carbohydrates: 23g

Protein: 5g

Sodium: 155mg

Almost Niçoise Salad

Difficulty Level: 2/5

Preparation time: 20 minutes

Cooking time: 5 minutes

Servings: 6

Ingredients:

1 pound small red potatoes, halved

8 ounces green beans, trimmed

1 head Boston lettuce, leaves separated

4 large hardboiled eggs, peeled and quartered (see tip)

8 cherry tomatoes, halved

¼ cup white wine vinegar

3 tablespoons Dijon mustard

⅛ teaspoon salt

⅛ teaspoon freshly ground black pepper

¼ cup olive oil

1 cup cured black olives

Directions:

Place the potatoes in a saucepan, cover with water, and bring to a boil over high heat. Cook for about 5 minutes until the potatoes are soft but not mushy. Drain and set aside.

In another saucepan over medium-high heat, heat enough water to cover the green beans until boiling. Add the green beans and cook for about 2 minutes to blanch.

Line shallow salad bowls with the lettuce leaves. Evenly divide the potatoes, green beans, egg quarters, and cherry tomatoes among the bowls.

In a small bowl, whisk the vinegar, mustard, salt, and pepper until combined. While whisking, slowly add the olive oil, until you have a well-emulsified dressing. Drizzle the dressing over the salads and top each with the olives before serving.

Nutrition:

Calories: 332

Total Fats: 21g

Saturated Fat: 4g

Fiber: 6g

Carbohydrates: 29g

Protein: 11g

Mediterranean Potato Salad

Difficulty Level: 2/5

Preparation time: 15 minutes

Cooking time: 15 minutes

Servings: 6

Ingredients:

4 russet potatoes

1 red bell pepper, seeded and finely diced

1 red onion, finely chopped

2 cups chopped fresh parsley

½ cup capers, drained

¼ cup olive oil

¼ cup freshly squeezed lemon juice

Grated zest of 1 lemon

1 teaspoon dried thyme

⅛ teaspoon salt

Directions:

Place the potatoes in a medium saucepan, cover with cold water, and bring to a boil over medium-high heat. Cook for about 15 minutes until the potatoes are soft but not overcooked. You want to be able to pierce them with a fork but have them stay whole. Drain and let cool.

Peel the potatoes and cut them into ½-inch cubes. Place the potatoes in a medium bowl.

Add the red bell pepper, red onion, parsley, and capers to the bowl and set aside.

In a small bowl, whisk the olive oil, lemon juice, lemon zest, thyme, and salt until well combined. Drizzle the dressing over the potato salad and toss until well coated. Serve chilled or at room temperature.

Nutrition:

Calories: 211

Total Fats: 9g

Saturated Fat: 1g

Fiber: 4g

Carbohydrates: 31g

Protein: 4g

Sodium: 312mg

Panzanella Salad

Difficulty Level: 2/5

Preparation time: 20 minutes

Cooking time: 5 minutes

Servings: 6

Ingredients:

1 small loaf French bread, cut into 1-inch cubes (about 6 cups)

¼ cup olive oil, divided

3 large tomatoes

2 Persian cucumbers, cut into ½-inch-thick rounds

1 small red onion, thinly sliced

1 cup chopped fresh basil

1 garlic clove, mashed to a paste

¼ cup red wine vinegar

⅛ teaspoon salt

Directions:

Preheat the oven to 350°F.

In a large bowl, toss the bread cubes with 2 tablespoons of olive oil until coated. Spread the cubes in a single layer on a baking sheet. Bake for 5 minutes or until the bread is lightly toasted. Divide the toasted cubes evenly among serving bowls.

Dice the tomatoes into a colander set over a bowl to collect the juices. Transfer the tomatoes to a medium bowl and set the bowl containing the juice aside.

Add the cucumbers, red onion, basil, and garlic to the tomatoes.

Add the remaining 2 tablespoons of olive oil, the vinegar, and salt to the bowl containing the tomato juice and whisk until well combined. Drizzle the dressing over the vegetables and toss well to mix.

Divide the vegetables and dressing among the bowls with the bread and serve.

Nutrition:

Calories: 348

Total Fats: 18g

Saturated Fat: 3g

Fiber: 3g

Carbohydrates: 41g

Protein: 8g

Sodium: 293mg

Lentil and Feta Salad

Difficulty Level: 2/5

Preparation time: 10 minutes

Cooking time: 15 minutes

Servings: 6

Ingredients:

2 cups chopped fresh parsley

2 celery stalks, diced

2 baby cucumbers, diced

1 red onion, diced

1 yellow bell pepper, seeded and diced

¼ cup olive oil

½ cup freshly squeezed lemon juice

1 teaspoon chopped fresh oregano

1 pound dried brown lentils, rinsed and picked over for debris

8 cups water

½ cup crumbled feta cheese

Directions:

In a large bowl, combine the parsley, celery, cucumbers, red onion, and yellow bell pepper. Set aside.

In a small bowl, whisk the olive oil, lemon juice, and oregano until well combined. Pour the dressing over the vegetables and toss well to coat. Set aside.

In a large pot over medium-high heat, combine the lentils and water. Bring to a boil. Once boiling, reduce the heat to maintain a simmer and cook for 15 minutes until the lentils are just done. Drain and add the lentils, while still hot, to the vegetables. Toss well to combine. Sprinkle with the feta cheese to serve.

Nutrition:

Calories: 402

Total Fats: 12g

Saturated Fat: 3g

Fiber: 25g

Carbohydrates: 52g

Protein: 23g

Sodium: 165mg

Greek Salad

Difficulty Level: 1/5

Preparation time: 20 minutes

Cooking time: 0 minutes

Servings: 6

Ingredients:

10 romaine lettuce leaves, chopped

1 red onion, thinly sliced

1 green bell pepper, seeded and chopped

2 large tomatoes, diced

2 Persian cucumbers, cut into slices

1 cup pitted Kalamata olives

¼ cup chopped fresh oregano

6 tablespoons olive oil

¼ cup freshly squeezed lemon juice

1 cup crumbled feta cheese

Directions:

In a large salad bowl, combine the lettuce leaves, red onion, green bell pepper, tomatoes, cucumbers, olives, and oregano. Toss until well mixed. Set aside.

In a small bowl, whisk the olive oil and lemon juice until blended. Pour the dressing over the salad and toss well to coat.

Sprinkle with the feta cheese to serve.

Nutrition:

Calories: 264

Total Fats: 22g

Saturated Fat: 6g

Fiber: 4g

Carbohydrates: 14g

Protein: 6g

Sodium: 342mg

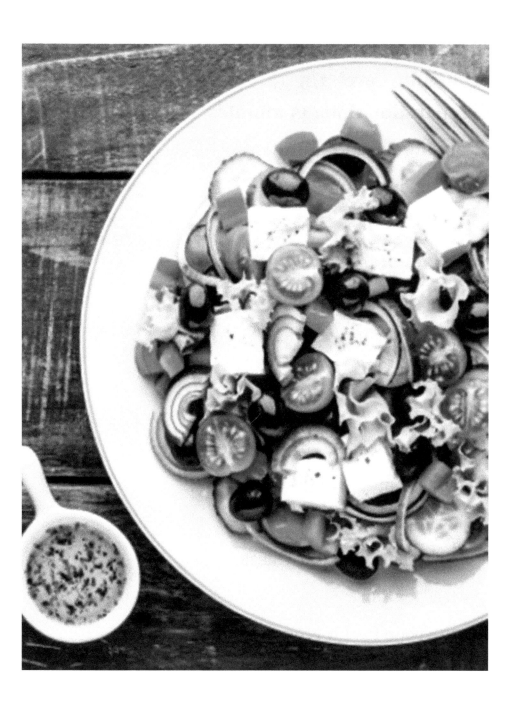

Shepherd's Salad

Difficulty Level: 1/5

Preparation time: 15 minutes

Cooking time: 0 minutes

Servings: 6

Ingredients:

4 large ripe tomatoes, diced

4 Persian cucumbers, diced

6 scallions, white and green parts, chopped

1 green bell pepper, seeded and chopped

1 cup crumbled feta cheese (optional)

½ cup chopped fresh parsley

¼ cup olive oil

3 tablespoons red wine vinegar

⅛ teaspoon salt

⅛ teaspoon freshly ground black pepper

Directions:

In a large salad bowl, combine the tomatoes, cucumbers, scallions, green bell pepper, feta cheese (if using), and parsley. Set aside.

In a small bowl, whisk the olive oil, vinegar, salt, and pepper until combined. Drizzle the dressing over the vegetables and toss well to coat.

Nutrition:

Calories: 139

Total Fats: 9g

Saturated Fat: 1g

Fiber: 3g

Carbohydrates: 15g

Protein: 3g

Sodium: 66mg

Spanish Green Beans

Difficulty Level: 2/5

Preparation time: 10 minutes

Cooking time: 20 minutes

Servings: 4

Ingredients:

¼ cup extra-virgin olive oil

1 large onion, chopped

4 cloves garlic, finely chopped

»1 pound green beans, fresh or frozen, trimmed

1½ teaspoons salt, divided

»1 (15-ounce) can diced tomatoes

½ teaspoon freshly ground black pepper

Directions:

In a large pot over medium heat, heat the olive oil, onion, and garlic; cook for 1 minute.

Cut the green beans into 2-inch pieces.

Add the green beans and 1 teaspoon of salt to the pot and toss everything together; cook for 3 minutes.

Add the diced tomatoes, remaining ½ teaspoon of salt, and black pepper to the pot; continue to cook for another 12 minutes, stirring occasionally.

Serve warm.

Nutrition:

Calories: 200;

Protein: 4g;

Total Carbohydrates: 18g;

Sugars: 9g;

Fiber: 6g;

Total Fat: 14g;

Saturated Fat: 2g;

Cholesterol: 0mg;

Sodium: 844mg

Rustic Cauliflower and Carrot Hash

Difficulty Level: 2/5

Preparation time: 10 minutes

Cooking time: 10 minutes

Servings: 4

Ingredients:

3 tablespoons extra-virgin olive oil

1 large onion, chopped

1 tablespoon garlic, minced

»2 cups carrots, diced

»4 cups cauliflower pieces, washed

1 teaspoon salt

»½ teaspoon ground cumin

Directions:

In a large skillet over medium heat, cook the olive oil, onion, garlic, and carrots for 3 minutes.

Cut the cauliflower into 1-inch or bite-size pieces. Add the cauliflower, salt, and cumin to the skillet and toss to combine with the carrots and onions.

Cover and cook for 3 minutes.

Toss the vegetables and continue to cook uncovered for an additional 3 to 4 minutes.

5. Serve warm.

Nutrition:

Calories: 159;

Protein: 3g;

Total Carbohydrates: 15g;

Sugars: 7g;

Fiber: 5g;

Total Fat: 11g;

Saturated Fat: 2g;

Cholesterol: 0mg;

Sodium: 657mg

Roasted Cauliflower and Tomatoes

Difficulty Level: 2/5

Preparation time: 25 minutes

Cooking time: 5 minutes

Servings: 4

Ingredients:

»4 cups cauliflower, cut into 1-inch pieces

6 tablespoons extra-virgin olive oil, divided

1 teaspoon salt, divided

»4 cups cherry tomatoes

½ teaspoon freshly ground black pepper

»½ cup grated Parmesan cheese

Directions:

Preheat the oven to 425°F.

Add the cauliflower, 3 tablespoons of olive oil, and ½ teaspoon of salt to a large bowl and toss to coat evenly. Pour onto a baking sheet and spread the cauliflower out in an even layer.

In another large bowl, add the tomatoes, remaining 3 tablespoons of olive oil, and ½ teaspoon of salt, and toss to coat evenly. Pour onto a different baking sheet.

Put the sheet of cauliflower and the sheet of tomatoes in the oven to roast for 17 to 20 minutes until the cauliflower is lightly browned and tomatoes are plump.

Using a spatula, spoon the cauliflower into a serving dish, and top with tomatoes, black pepper, and Parmesan cheese. Serve warm.

Nutrition:

Calories: 294;

Protein: 9g;

Total Carbohydrates: 13g;

Sugars: 6g;

Fiber: 4g;

Total Fat: 26g;

Saturated Fat: 6g;

Cholesterol: 10mg;

Sodium: 858mg

Sautéed Garlic Spinach

Difficulty Level: 2/5

Preparation time: 5 minutes

Cooking time: 10 minutes

Servings: 4

Ingredients:

¼ cup extra-virgin olive oil

1 large onion, thinly sliced

3 cloves garlic, minced

»6 (1-pound) bags of baby spinach, washed

½ teaspoon salt

»1 lemon, cut into wedges

Directions:

Cook the olive oil, onion, and garlic in a large skillet for 2 minutes over medium heat.

Add one bag of spinach and ½ teaspoon of salt. Cover the skillet and let the spinach wilt for 30 seconds. Repeat (omitting the salt), adding 1 bag of spinach at a time.

Once all the spinach has been added, remove the cover and cook for 3 minutes, letting some of the moisture evaporate.

Serve warm with a generous squeeze of lemon over the top.

Nutrition:

Calories: 301;

Protein: 17g;

Total Carbohydrates: 29g;

Sugars: 2g;

Fiber: 17g;

Total Fat: 14g;

Saturated Fat: 2g;

Cholesterol: 0mg;

Sodium: 812mg

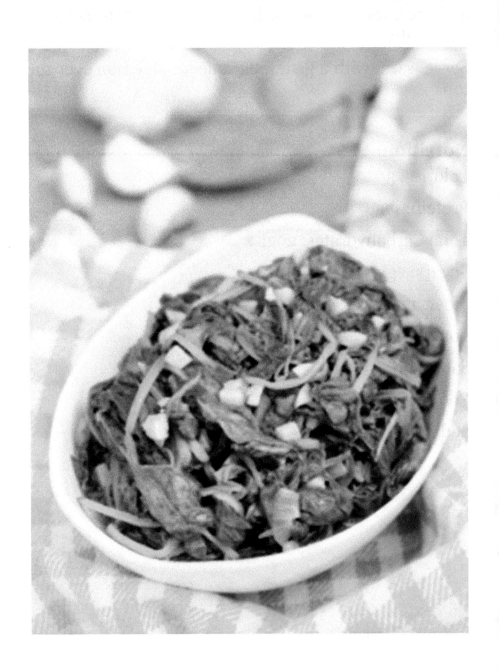

Garlicky Sautéed Zucchini with Mint

Difficulty Level: 2/5

Preparation time: 5 minutes

Cooking time: 10 minutes

Servings: 4

Ingredients:

»3 large green zucchini

3 tablespoons extra-virgin olive oil

1 large onion, chopped

3 cloves garlic, minced

1 teaspoon salt

»1 teaspoon dried mint

Directions:

Cut the zucchini into ½-inch cubes.

In a large skillet over medium heat, cook the olive oil, onions, and garlic for 3 minutes, stirring constantly.

Add the zucchini and salt to the skillet and toss to combine with the onions and garlic, cooking for 5 minutes.

Add the mint to the skillet, tossing to combine. Cook for another 2 minutes. Serve warm.

Nutrition:

Calories: 147;

Protein: 4g;

Total Carbohydrates: 12g;

Sugars: 6g;

Fiber: 3g;

Total Fat: 11g;

Saturated Fat: 2g;

Cholesterol: 0mg;

Sodium: 607mg

Stewed Okra

Difficulty Level: 2/5

Preparation time: 5 minutes

Cooking time: 25 minutes

Servings: 4

Ingredients:

¼ cup extra-virgin olive oil

1 large onion, chopped

4 cloves garlic, finely chopped

1 teaspoon salt

»1 pound fresh or frozen okra, cleaned

»1 (15-ounce) can plain tomato sauce

2 cups water

»½ cup fresh cilantro, finely chopped

½ teaspoon freshly ground black pepper

Directions:

In a large pot over medium heat, stir and cook the olive oil, onion, garlic, and salt for 1 minute.

Stir in the okra and cook for 3 minutes.

Add the tomato sauce, water, cilantro, and black pepper; stir, cover, and let cook for 15 minutes, stirring occasionally.

Serve warm.

Nutrition:

Calories: 201;

Protein: 4g;

Total Carbohydrates: 18g;

Sugars: 8g;

Fiber: 6g;

Total Fat: 14g;

Saturated Fat: 2g;

Cholesterol: 0mg;

Sodium: 1,156mg

Fava and Garbanzo Bean Fūl

Difficulty Level: 2/5

Preparation time: 10 minutes

Cooking time: 10 minutes

Servings: 6

Ingredients:

»1 (16-ounce) can garbanzo beans, rinsed and drained

»1 (15-ounce) can fava beans, rinsed and drained

3 cups water

½ cup lemon juice

3 cloves garlic, peeled and minced

1 teaspoon salt

3 tablespoons extra-virgin olive oil

Directions:

In a 3-quart pot over medium heat, cook the garbanzo beans, fava beans, and water for 10 minutes.

Reserving 1 cup of the liquid from the cooked beans, drain the beans and put them in a bowl.

Mix the reserved liquid, lemon juice, minced garlic, and salt together and add to the beans in the bowl. Using a potato masher, mash up about half the beans in the bowl.

After mashing half the beans, give the mixture one more stir to make sure the beans are evenly mixed.

Drizzle the olive oil over the top.

Serve warm or cold with pita bread.

Nutrition:

Calories: 199;

Protein: 10g;

Total Carbohydrates: 25g;

Sugars: 4g;

Fiber: 9g;

Total Fat: 9g;

Saturated Fat: 1g;

Cholesterol: 0mg;

Sodium: 395mg

Confetti Couscous

Difficulty Level: 2/5

Preparation time: 5 minutes

Cooking time: 20 minutes

Servings: 4-6

Ingredients:

3 tablespoons extra-virgin olive oil

1 large onion, chopped

»2 carrots, chopped

»1 cup fresh peas

»½ cup golden raisins

1 teaspoon salt

»2 cups vegetable broth

»2 cups couscous

Directions:

In a medium pot over medium heat, gently toss the olive oil, onions, carrots, peas, and raisins together and let cook for 5 minutes.

Add the salt and broth, and stir to combine. Bring to a boil, and let ingredients boil for 5 minutes.

Add the couscous. Stir, turn the heat to low, cover, and let cook for 10 minutes. Fluff with a fork and serve.

Nutrition:

Calories: 511;

Protein: 14g;

Total Carbohydrates: 92g;

Sugars: 17g;

Fiber: 7g;

Total Fat: 12g;

Saturated Fat: 2g;

Cholesterol: 0mg;

Sodium: 504mg

Lemon Orzo with Fresh Herbs

Difficulty Level: 2/5

Preparation time: 10 minutes

Cooking time: 10 minutes

Servings: 4

Ingredients:

»2 cups orzo

½ cup fresh parsley, finely chopped

½ cup fresh basil, finely chopped

»2 tablespoons lemon zest

½ cup extra-virgin olive oil

⅓ cup lemon juice

1 teaspoon salt

½ teaspoon freshly ground black pepper

Directions:

Bring a large pot of water to a boil. Add the orzo and cook for 7 minutes. Drain and rinse with cold water. Let the orzo sit in a strainer to drain and cool completely.

Once the orzo has cooled, put it in a large bowl and add the parsley, basil, and lemon zest.

In a small bowl, whisk together the olive oil, lemon juice, salt, and pepper. Add the dressing to the pasta and toss everything together. Serve at room temperature or chilled.

Nutrition:

Calories: 568;

Protein: 11g;

Total Carbohydrates: 65g;

Sugars: 4g;

Fiber: 4g;

Total Fat: 29g;

Saturated Fat: 4g;

Cholesterol: 0mg;

Sodium: 586mg

Orzo-Veggie Pilaf

Difficulty Level: 2/5

Preparation time: 20 minutes

Cooking time: 10 minutes

Servings: 6

Ingredients:

»2 cups orzo

»1 pint (2 cups) cherry tomatoes, cut in half

»1 cup Kalamata olives

½ cup fresh basil, finely chopped

½ cup extra-virgin olive oil

»⅓ cup balsamic vinegar

1 teaspoon salt

½ teaspoon freshly ground black pepper

Directions:

Bring a large pot of water to a boil. Add the orzo and cook for 7 minutes. Drain and rinse the orzo with cold water in a strainer.

Once the orzo has cooled, put it in a large bowl. Add the tomatoes, olives, and basil.

In a small bowl, whisk together the olive oil, vinegar, salt, and pepper. Add this dressing to the pasta and toss everything together. Serve at room temperature or chilled.

Nutrition:

Calories: 476;

Protein: 8g;

Total Carbohydrates: 48g;

Sugars: 3g;

Fiber: 3g;

Total Fat: 28g;

Saturated Fat: 4g;

Cholesterol: 0mg;

Sodium: 851mg

Bulgur and Garbanzo Pilaf

Difficulty Level: 2/5

Preparation time: 5 minutes

Cooking time: 20 minutes

Servings: 4-6

Ingredients:

3 tablespoons extra-virgin olive oil

1 large onion, chopped

»1 (16-ounce) can garbanzo beans, rinsed and drained

»2 cups bulgur wheat #3, rinsed and drained

1½ teaspoons salt

»½ teaspoon cinnamon

4 cups water

Directions:

In a large pot over medium heat, cook the olive oil and onion for 5 minutes.

Add the garbanzo beans and cook for another 5 minutes.

Add the bulgur, salt, cinnamon, and water and stir to combine. Cover the pot, turn the heat to low, and cook for 10 minutes.

When the cooking is done, fluff the pilaf with a fork. Cover and let sit for another 5 minutes.

Nutrition:

Calories: 462;

Protein: 15g;

Total Carbohydrates: 76g;

Sugars: 5g;

Fiber: 19g;

Total Fat: 13g;

Saturated Fat: 2g;

Cholesterol: 0mg;

Sodium: 890mg

Spanish Rice

Difficulty Level: 2/5

Preparation time:10 minutes

Cooking time: 20 minutes

Servings: 4

Ingredients:

2 tablespoons extra-virgin olive oil

1 medium onion, finely chopped

»1 large tomato, finely diced

»2 tablespoons tomato paste

»1 teaspoon smoked paprika

1 teaspoon salt

»1½ cups basmati rice

3 cups water

Directions:

In a medium pot over medium heat, cook the olive oil, onion, and tomato for 3 minutes.

Stir in the tomato paste, paprika, salt, and rice. Cook for 1 minute.

Add the water, cover the pot, and turn the heat to low. Cook for 12 minutes.

Gently toss the rice, cover, and cook for another 3 minutes.

Nutrition:

Calories: 328;

Protein: 6g;

Total Carbohydrates: 60g;

Sugars: 3g;

Fiber: 2g;

Total Fat: 7g;

Saturated Fat: 1g;

Cholesterol: 0mg;

Sodium: 651mg

Garbanzo and Pita No-Bake Casserole

Difficulty Level: 2/5

Preparation time: 10 minutes

Cooking time: 10 minutes

Servings: 4

Ingredients:
»4 cups Greek yogurt

3 cloves garlic, minced

1 teaspoon salt

»2 (16-ounce) cans garbanzo beans, rinsed and drained

2 cups water

»4 cups pita chips

»5 tablespoons unsalted butter

Directions:

In a large bowl, whisk together the yogurt, garlic, and salt. Set aside.

Put the garbanzo beans and water in a medium pot. Bring to a boil; let beans boil for about 5 minutes.

Pour the garbanzo beans and the liquid into a large casserole dish.

Top the beans with pita chips. Pour the yogurt sauce over the pita chip layer.

In a small saucepan, melt and brown the butter, about 3 minutes. Pour the brown butter over the yogurt sauce.

Nutrition:

Calories: 772;

Protein: 39g;

Total Carbohydrates: 73g;

Sugars: 18g;

Fiber: 13g;

Total Fat: 36g;

Saturated Fat: 15g;

Cholesterol: 71mg;

Sodium: 1,003mg

Quick Shrimp Fettuccine

Difficulty Level: 2/5

Preparation time: 10 minutes

Cooking time: 10 minutes

Servings: 4-6

Ingredients:
»8 ounces fettuccine pasta

¼ cup extra-virgin olive oil

3 tablespoons garlic, minced

»1 pound large shrimp (21-25), peeled and deveined

⅓ cup lemon juice

»1 tablespoon lemon zest

½ teaspoon salt

½ teaspoon freshly ground black pepper

Directions:

Bring a large pot of salted water to a boil. Add the fettuccine and cook for 8 minutes.

In a large saucepan over medium heat, cook the olive oil and garlic for 1 minute.

Add the shrimp to the saucepan and cook for 3 minutes on each side. Remove the shrimp from the pan and set aside.

Add the lemon juice and lemon zest to the saucepan, along with the salt and pepper.

Reserve ½ cup of the pasta water and drain the pasta.

Add the pasta water to the saucepan with the lemon juice and zest and stir everything together. Add the pasta and toss together to coat the pasta evenly. Transfer the pasta to a serving dish and top with the cooked shrimp. Serve warm.

Nutrition:

Calories: 615;

Protein: 33g;

Total Carbohydrates: 89g;

Sugars: 3g;

Fiber: 4g;

Total Fat: 17g;

Saturated Fat: 2g;

Cholesterol: 145mg;

Sodium: 407mg

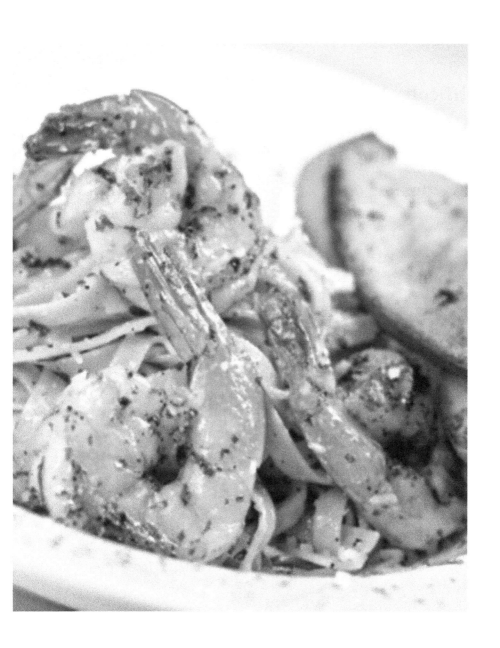

White Pizza with Prosciutto and Arugula

Difficulty Level: 2/5

Preparation time: 10 minutes

Cooking time: 15 minutes

Servings: 4

Ingredients:

»1 pound prepared pizza dough

»½ cup ricotta cheese

1 tablespoon garlic, minced

»1 cup grated mozzarella cheese

»3 ounces prosciutto, thinly sliced

½ cup fresh arugula

½ teaspoon freshly ground black pepper

Directions:

Preheat the oven to 450°F. Roll out the pizza dough on a floured surface.

Put the pizza dough on a parchment-lined baking sheet or pizza sheet. Put the dough in the oven and bake for 8 minutes.

In a small bowl, mix together the ricotta, garlic, and mozzarella.

Remove the pizza dough from the oven and spread the cheese mixture over the top. Bake for another 5 to 6 minutes.

Top the pizza with prosciutto, arugula, and pepper; serve warm.

Nutrition:

Calories: 435;

Protein: 20g;

Total Carbohydrates: 51g;

Sugars: 0g;

Fiber: 4g;

Total Fat: 17g;

Saturated Fat: 8g;

Cholesterol: 53mg;

Sodium: 1,630mg

9 781802 774511

WE CAN READ
AND WRITE
Book 2

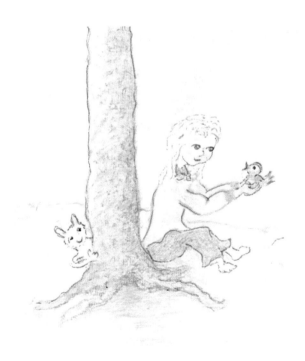

Trudy Dorn

Author and Illustrator

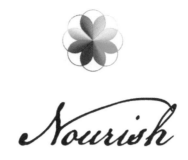

Nourish

The author and publisher invite

not-for-profit reproduction and sharing

of this book for educational or learning purposes.

Published by Nourish Publishing

West Vancouver, BC Canada.

ISBN: 9781777361716

NOURISH.press

Learn more about the author at:

TrudyDorn.net

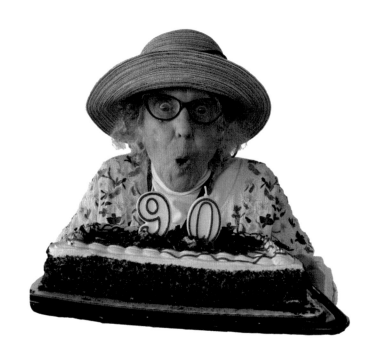

We Can Read and Write, Book 2,
is the second of Grandma Trudy's books.

She wrote and illustrated these books to help
children and adults around the world
to learn English.

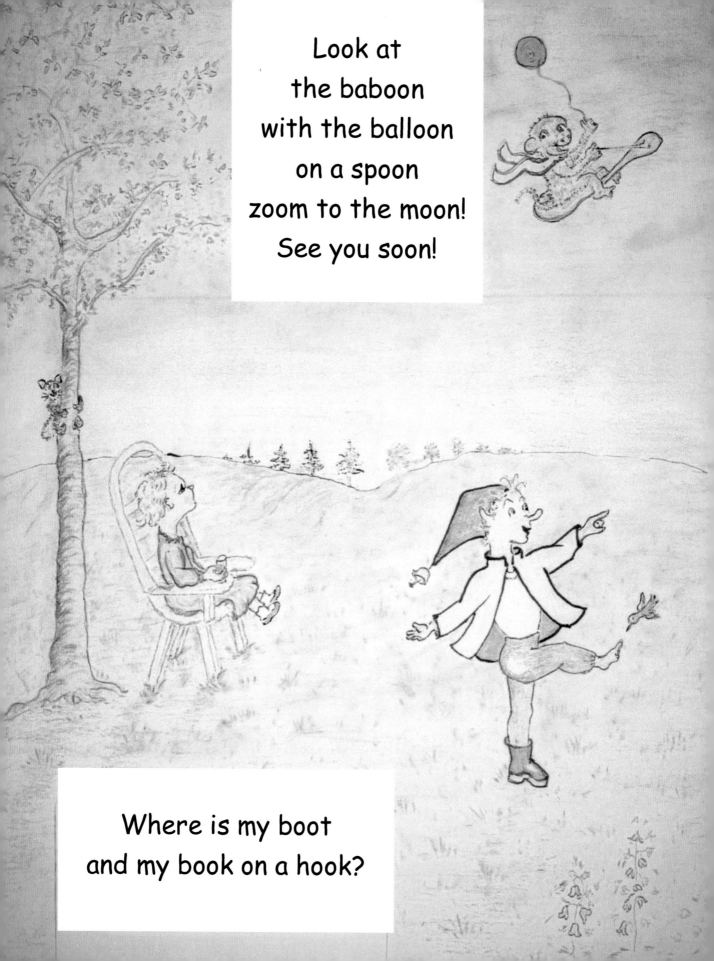

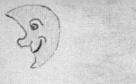

We zoom to the zoo.
"Cool man, cool!"
said the goose on the moose.

We are in a good mood.

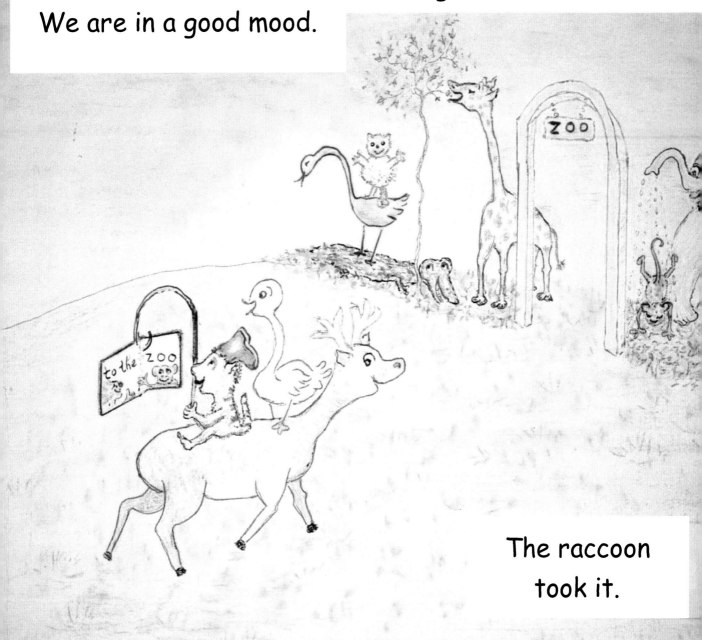

The raccoon
took it.

The boot is on his head.
"He took the book too,"
said the goose on the moose.

The cook cooks good food.
It is good!

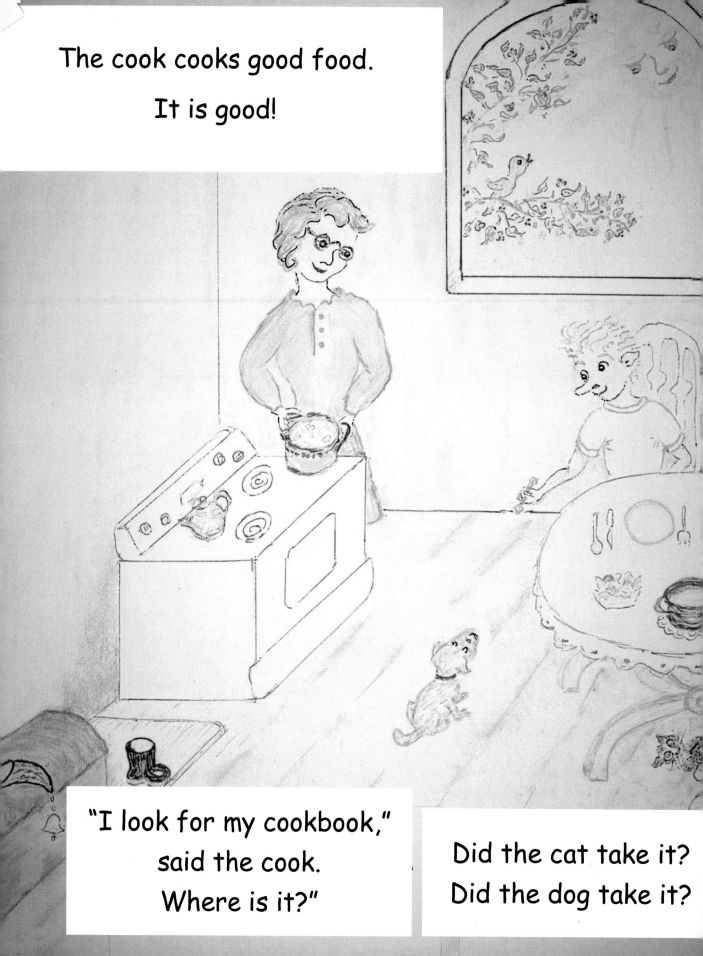

"I look for my cookbook,"
said the cook.
Where is it?"

Did the cat take it?
Did the dog take it?

"We zoom to the zoo,"
said the goose on the moose.
"Raccoon, there is room for you."

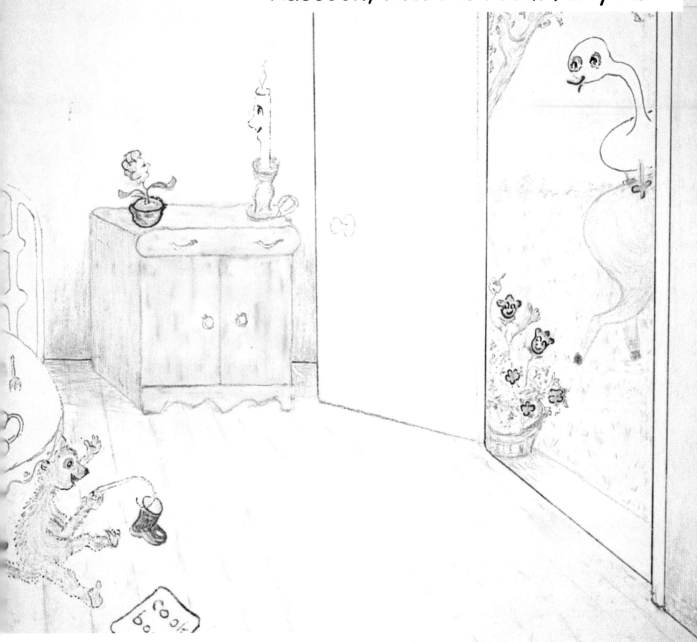

The raccoon took it.
Your cookbook is with
the raccoon.

Look, he took a hook,
a boot and a book too.

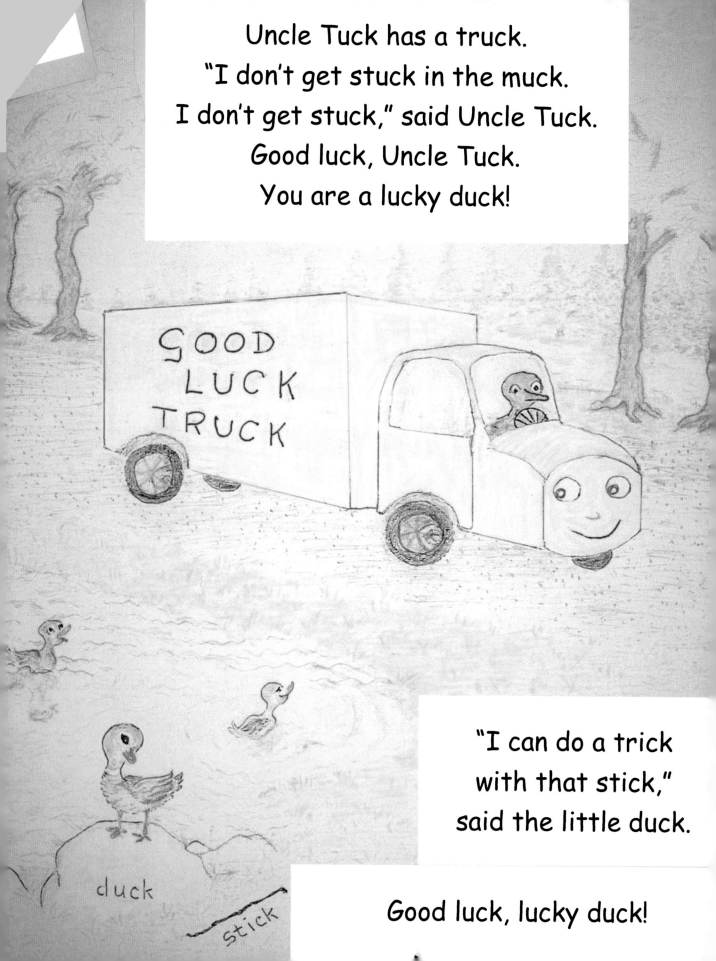

Uncle Tuck has a truck.
"I don't get stuck in the muck.
I don't get stuck," said Uncle Tuck.
Good luck, Uncle Tuck.
You are a lucky duck!

"I can do a trick
with that stick,"
said the little duck.

Good luck, lucky duck!

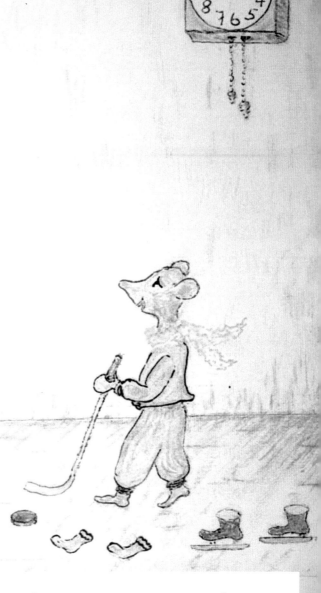

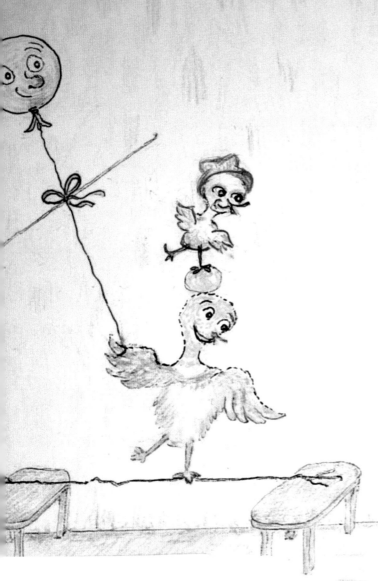

See my trick
on my stick?

"Tick tock," said the clock.
"I see your sock."

Where are my socks?
I play hockey
with my hockey stick.

Here is the alphabet with its 26 letters:

a – b – c – d – e – f – g –
h – i – j – k – l – m – n – o – p –
q – r – s – t – u – v – w – x – y – z

We begin a new sentence with a capital letter. We also use a capital letter for the first letter of a name. Here are the capital letters of the alphabet:

A – B – C – D – E – F – G –
H – I – J – K – L – M – N – O – P –
Q – R – S – T – U – V – W – X – Y – Z

Some people like to write with cursive letters:

a b c d e f g h i
j k l m n o p q r
s t u v w x y z

Cursive capital letters are:

A - B - C - D - E - F - G
H - I - J - K - L - M - N
O - P - Q - R - S - T - U
V - W - X - Y - Z.

Try writing these letter on your own paper.

ape, the elephant, the Inca, the octopus and the ugly ling were sad.

Their names all start with a vowel.

The vowels are a, e, i, o, u and sometimes y.

When the word "a" is in front of a word with a vowel, you have to change the "a" to "an".

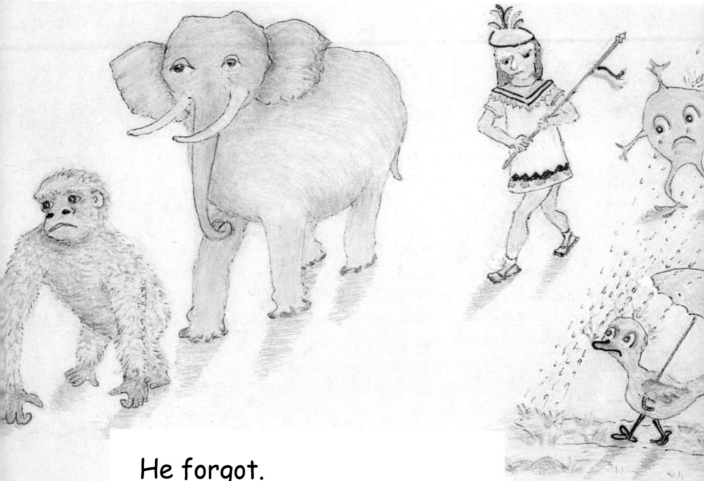

He forgot.

He wrote "a ape."

That is not correct!

Now an ape is sad,

and the others are too.

An eagle came by,
out of an open sky.
He had the "n" for all of them.

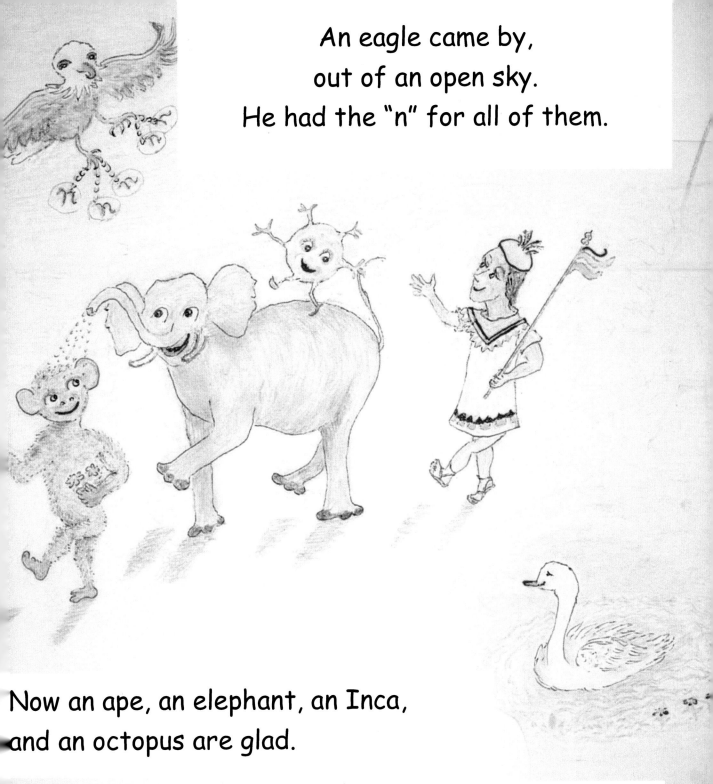

Now an ape, an elephant, an Inca,
and an octopus are glad.

An ugly duckling was so happy,
he changed into an artistic swan.

Queen Quick questions Quack-Quack.
She gives Quack-Quack a quarter
and a square to a squirrel.

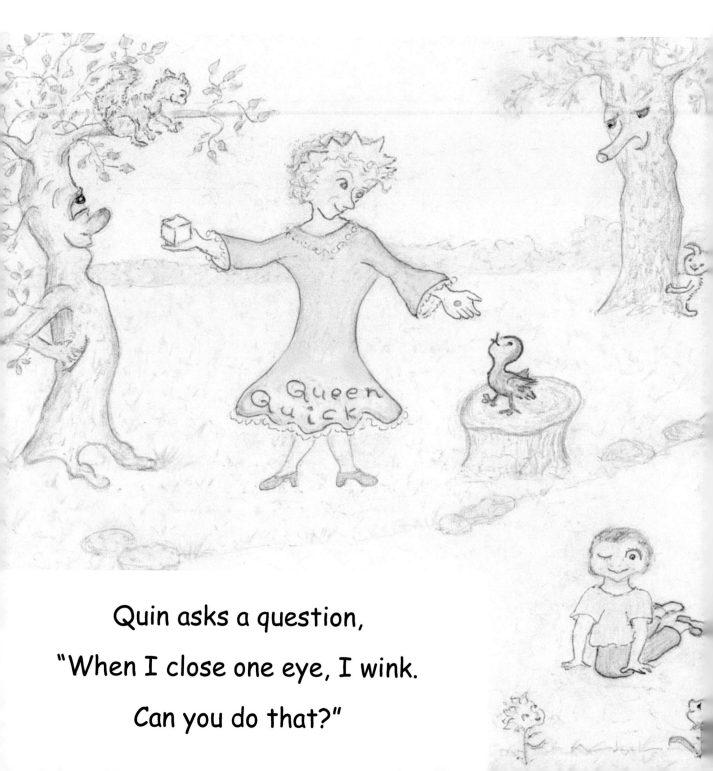

Quin asks a question,
"When I close one eye, I wink.
Can you do that?"

Quack-Quack went to Quebec.

She wanted to square dance with a squirrel.

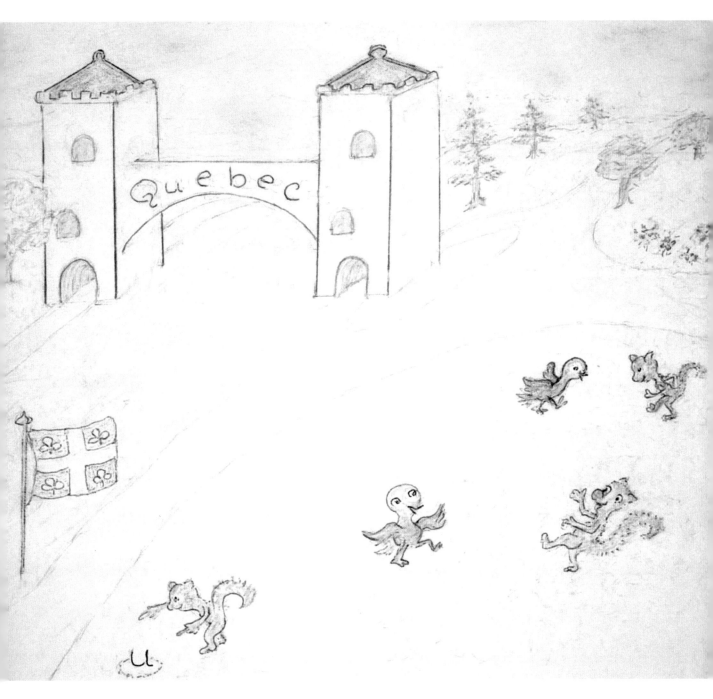

This squeaky squirrel has to go back quickly.

He forgot there is always a "u" after a "q."

A clown from downtown
asked a cow, who was all brown,
"Have you seen my crown?"

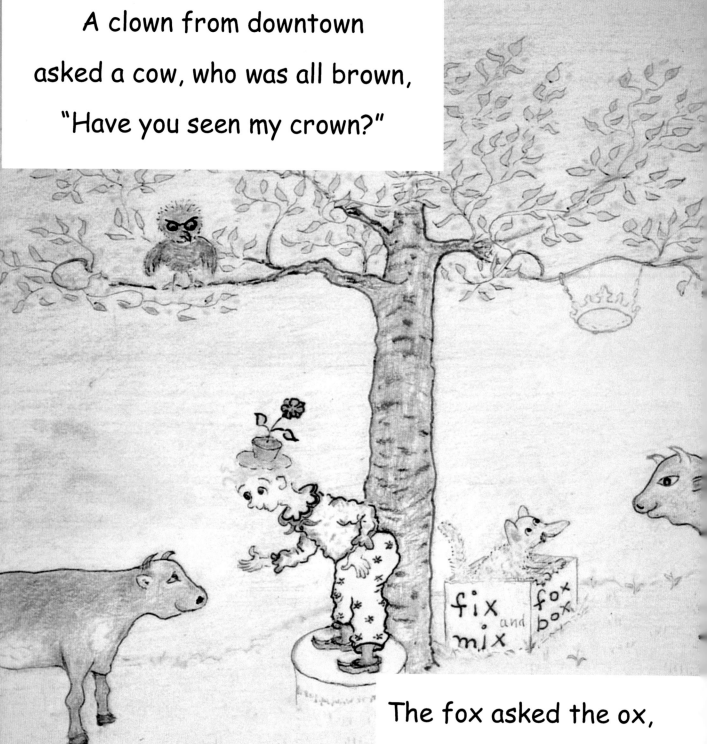

The fox asked the ox,
"How do we fix this box?"

The cow said, "Ask the owl."

The owl said, "Ask the ox."

The ox said, "Ask the fox."

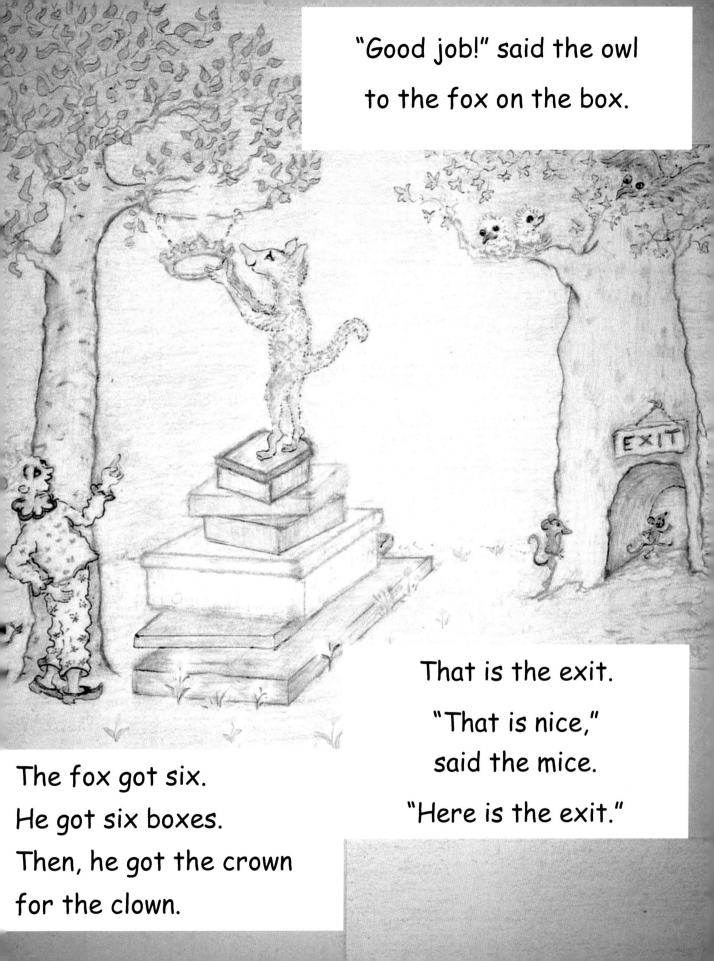

"Good job!" said the owl
to the fox on the box.

That is the exit.

"That is nice,"
said the mice.

"Here is the exit."

The fox got six.
He got six boxes.
Then, he got the crown
for the clown.

A fairy with golden hair sits on a chair and holds a ring of gold.

She is beautiful

and as sweet as pure sugar.

fairy tale
land

"Sure, I used to hear music.
It was a happy tune,"
the unicorn said.
"There is beauty in music."

Big bear had a pear in his hand.
There was bread on the table
in the meadow.
Is it heavy?
No, it is pleasant,
a little bit of heaven.

"My nose knows this is a rose,"
said the mole in a hole.

bear

in
bear
heaven

bread

mole
hill

The mole said: "I am told I am so old.
I hope I can go over those stones."

No, don't go in those holes.
It is cold in that whole hole.
I told you so.

We see a bee between three green trees,
and he sees me.
Sweet little bee, is your honey free?

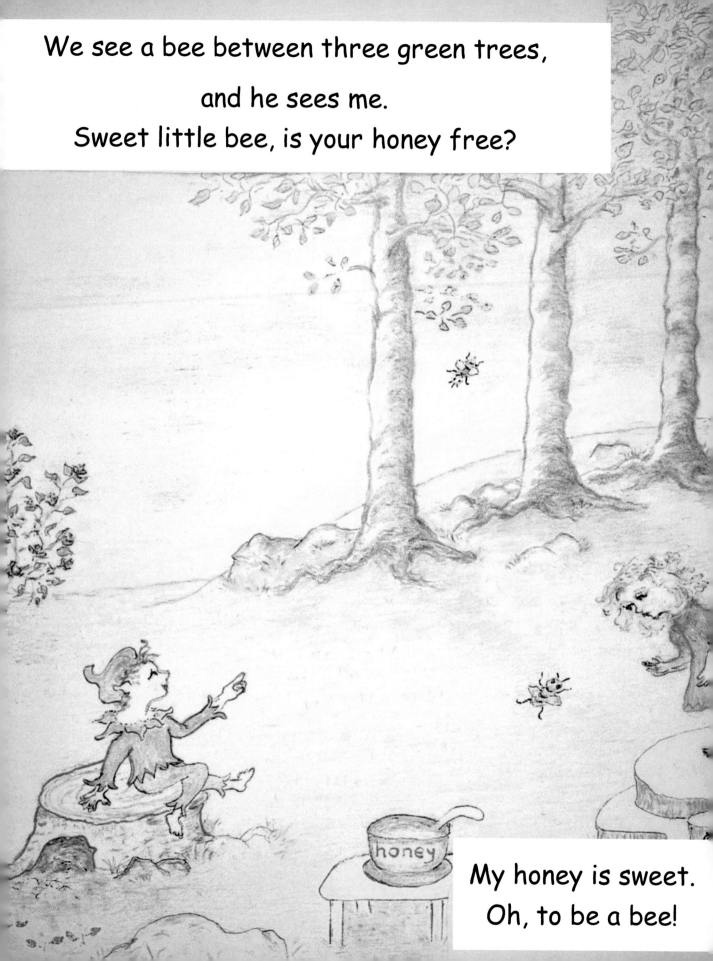

My honey is sweet.
Oh, to be a bee!

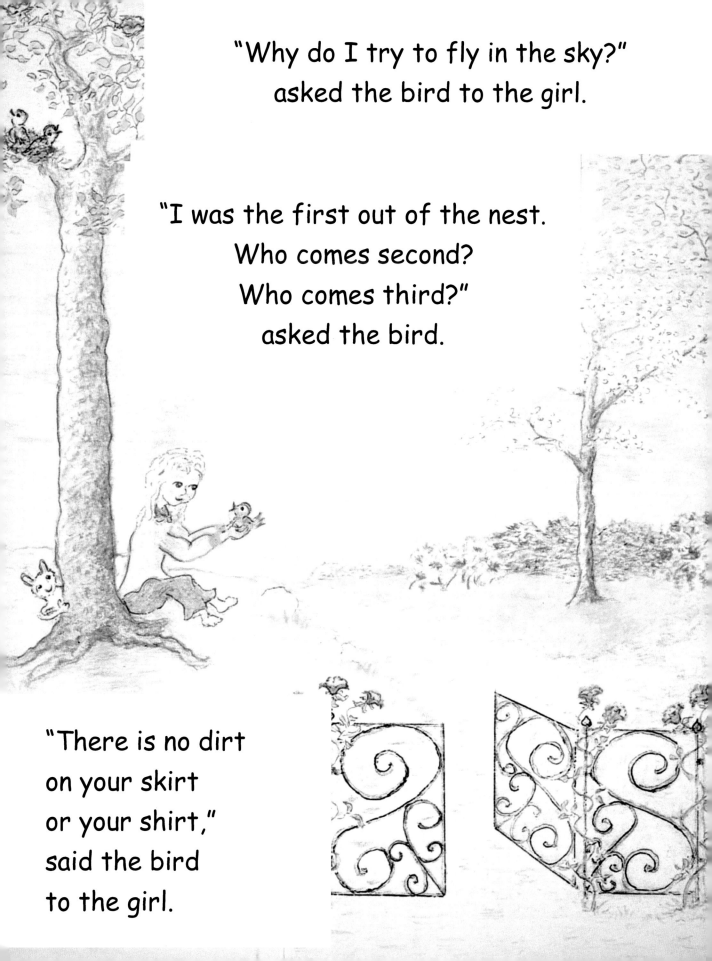

"Why do I try to fly in the sky?"
asked the bird to the girl.

"I was the first out of the nest.
Who comes second?
Who comes third?"
asked the bird.

"There is no dirt
on your skirt
or your shirt,"
said the bird
to the girl.

All the tall
and also the small
swans
saw the ball fall
over the wall.

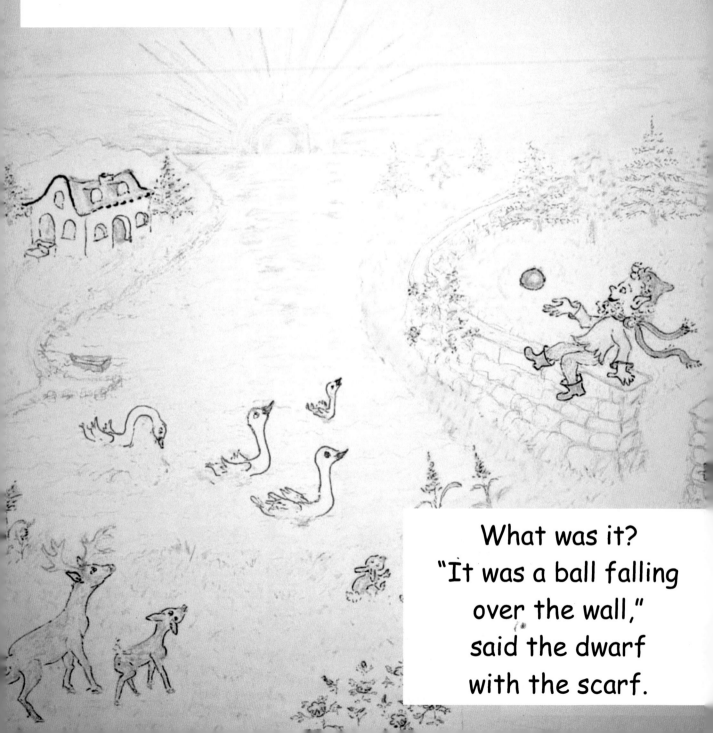

What was it?
"It was a ball falling
over the wall,"
said the dwarf
with the scarf.

It was dark in the park.

We want to talk.

We want to walk.

What is the glowing heart doing near the wall?

"I saw a saw on a log," said the frog.

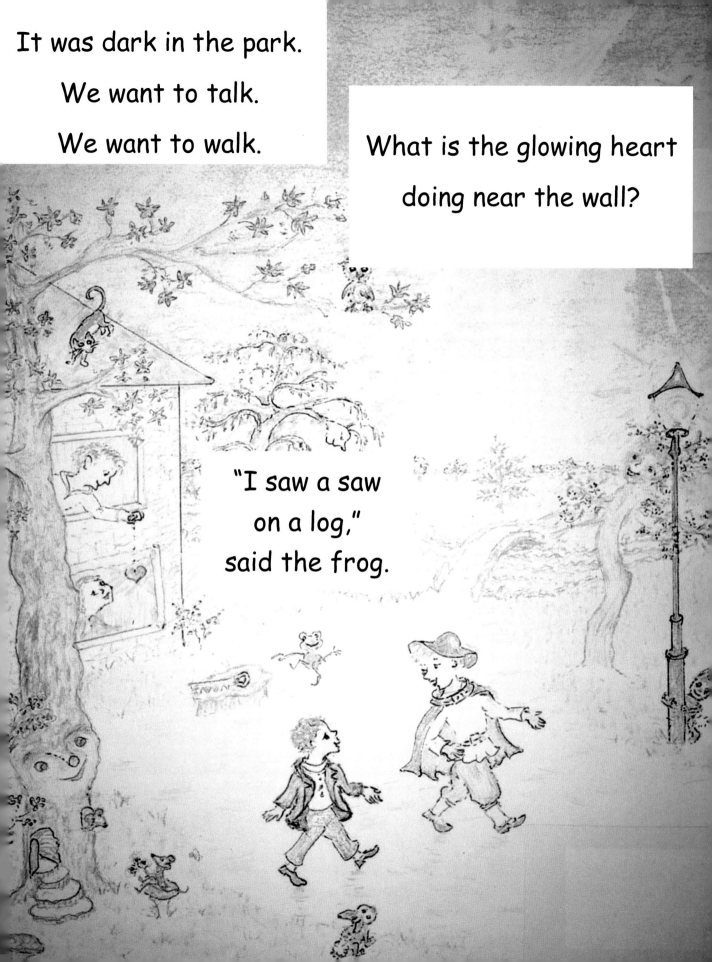

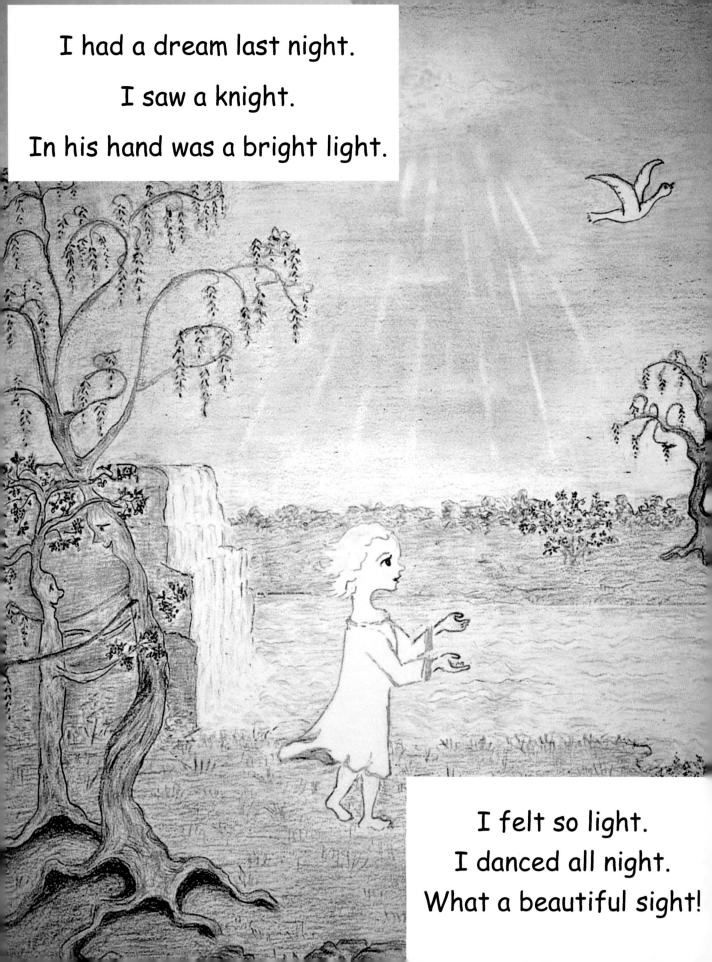

I had a dream last night.
I saw a knight.
In his hand was a bright light.

I felt so light.
I danced all night.
What a beautiful sight!

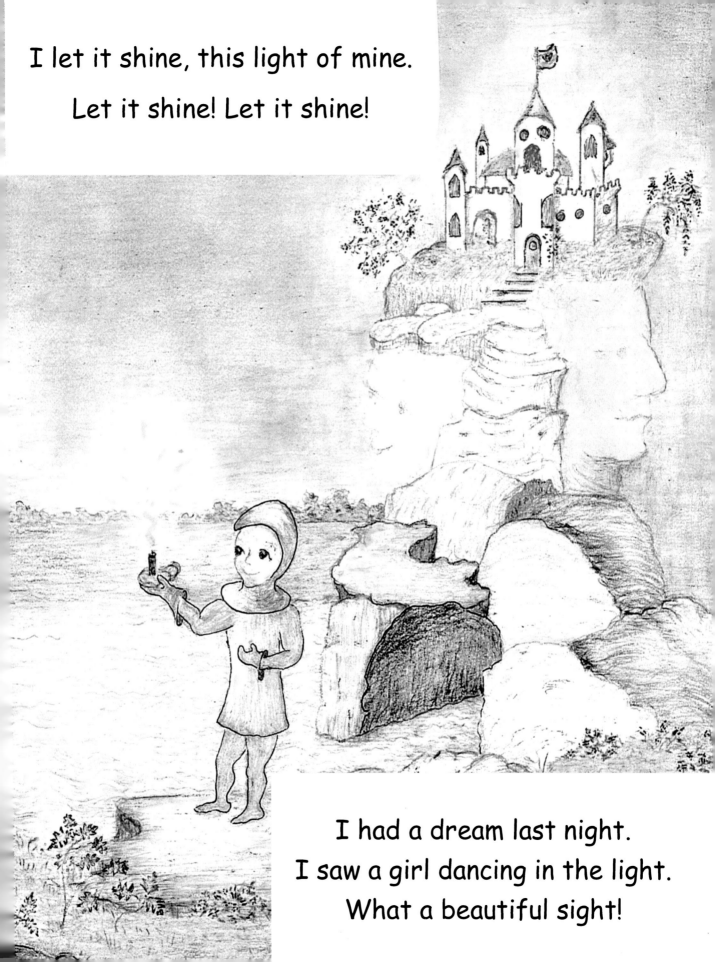

I let it shine, this light of mine.
Let it shine! Let it shine!

I had a dream last night.
I saw a girl dancing in the light.
What a beautiful sight!

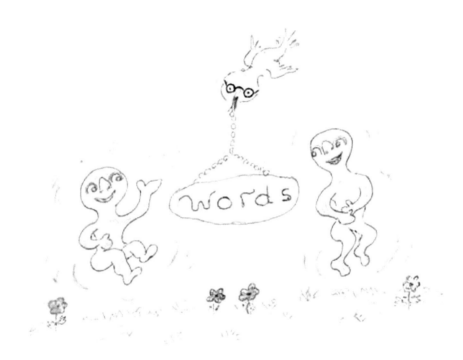

Sounds of Special Letters

You can write sentences with these words and draw nice pictures too.

oo

look – book – hook – took – foot –
good – wood – wool – wolf – wolves – cook –
cookies – bloom

Words with "oo" but sound differently from above:

boot – loot – root – moon – baboon – spoon –
soon – raccoon – tool – fool – cool – zoo –
food – mood – goose – loose – moose – zoom –
true – blue – glue – fruit – juice –
two (= 2) – to – too (= also) – do – super –
you – soup – through – prune – rule

Try these sentences:
Two raccoons looked to the moon too.
Two wolves zoom to the zoo too.
You do that too?

ck

luck – duck – truck – stuck – muck

back – pack

neck

stick – prick – trick – sick – pick

sock – hockey – hockey stick –

clock – tick-tock – rock – rocky

puck

Try three sentences:

My uncle had a pack on his back.

He picked up a pack of socks with a stick.

He was lucky!

Capital letters

Always begin a new sentence with a capital letter.

Names of people, places, and countries start with a capital letter.

Example: In America and in Canada, we write letters to John.

We do not write: "in america and canada, we write letters to john."

Oh boy! That last sentence has no capital letters. Oops!

Here is another sentence:

He writes a letter to an American and a Canadian.

Why is "an" in front of "American" and not in front of "Canadian"? Because the word "American" starts with a <u>vowel</u> and the word "Canadian" starts with a <u>consonant</u>.

an

When a word starts with a vowel, then instead of putting "a" in front of it you put "an." Here are some words that begin with a vowel. Can you make a sentence with some of these words in it?

an animal – an ape – an eagle – an alligator – an ant – an American – an apple – an aunt – an uncle – an egg – an elf – an entrance – an exit – an extra – an elephant – an ox – an old – an open – an orange – an intelligent – an interesting – an island – an itch – an umbrella – an underdog

Here are some examples:

An eagle said to an alligator, "I can't find an orange Easter egg."

An elephant came to help, but he could not find it. Then came an ant. He went on an adventure trip and found the orange egg under an umbrella.

An ape lifted an arm, "Hurrah! Even if you are small, you can help." Then the ant got an extra ride on an alligator to an amusement park.

qu

qua

quake – quality – quantity – quarrel – quartz – quarter = one quart (= $\frac{1}{4}$) – 4 quarters (= one dollar) – aquarium (aqua = water in Latin) – Squamish – square

que

plaque – queen – question – request – squeeze – Quebec – conquer – technique – frequency – unique

qui

quick – quiz – require – quiet – quite – squirrel – squint

The quick question is: "Did the squirrel squeeze the queen in the aquarium?"

OW

how – now – cow – vow – bow – allow –
towel – clown – brown – frown – down – town –
cowboy – coward – owl – howl –
WOW!

X

exit – exam – example – exercise –
excel – excellent – except – exciting – excuse –
export – expire – explain – explore – extra

six – mix – fix
box – fox – ox

Try these sentences:
Now, how did the clown go downtown with a cow?
The fox fixed a box and jumped on an ox.

u

music – use – useful – cucumber –
cute – unity – university
pure – cure – sure

The "ew" vowel sound sounds like the letter "u":
new – I knew – dew – fruit – juice – beautiful –
you – true – blue – glue – flute
through – soup

ai

fair – fairy – hair – chair – stairs – air – a pair

o

rose – nose – no – over – those – stones –
alone – open – only – below – I know – he knows –
hope – home – a hole – a whole hole –
blow – row – bow – arrow – flow – snow –
I know – he knows

ea

heaven – bear – pear – bread – head – pleasant

Try these sentences:

My nose knows this is a rose.

The bear put a pear on his head instead of his bread.

ou

I could – I should – I would

ey / ee

honey – money – monkey – donkey

I see – he sees – a bee

i

girl – bird – first – third –
dirt – shirt – skirt – stir – thirst – thirsty –
fir tree – birth – birthday

u

hurt – burn – purse – purple
run – under – sun – bun – uncle – fun

Try these sentences:
The third girl with the purple shirt learns to run
to the first fir tree. She earned a medal.
And she had a birthday party. It was fun!
Oh, to be a bee. My honey is free.
"That honey costs no money," said the monkey to the donkey.

a

what – was – arm – harm – sharp – wash – wallet –
awe – awestruck – charm – chalk – car – carnival
water – scarf – salt – spark – harmony –
saw – raw – law – paw – garden – hard –
all – tall – small – ball – fall – wall – call –
swan – dawn – lawn – fawn – car – sharp –
I want – he wants – I walk – he walks – watch
warm – quarter – dwarf

Try these sentences:
What was the dwarf doing on the wall?
He wanted to watch a ball fall into warm water.
Who saw the saw in the dark of the park?
A frog saw it. He danced around.
My friend walked with me and he talked with me.
There was a spark in the dark.

ed

*To describe actions in the past, most verbs (action words)
have "ed" added to the end.*

Examples: talk → talked, walk → walked, move → moved

But some words do not follow this rule. Examples:

know → knew – write → wrote – see → saw – do → did –
read → read – stand → stood – tell → told – sell → sold –
think → thought – bring → brought – buy → bought –
go → went – catch → caught – teach → taught –
eat → ate – stand → stood – find → found – is → was

silent "k" and "gh"

Some words begin with "k" but you don't hear "k."

knight – knife – I know – I knew – knack – knock – knob
– knot – knee

Some words have "gh" in it, but you don't hear that "gh"

light – night – sight – bright – fright – height – tight
laugh – cough – thought

Try this sentence: In the night the moonlight was bright.

Made in the USA
Monee, IL
31 October 2020